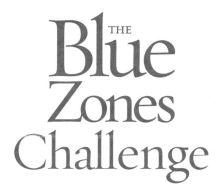

THE
Blue
Zones
Challenge

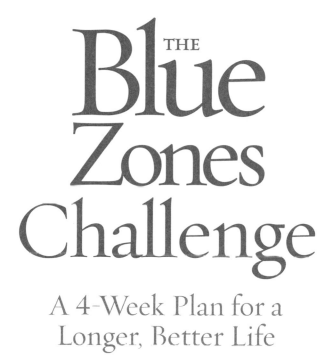

THE
Blue Zones Challenge

A 4-Week Plan for a
Longer, Better Life

DAN BUETTNER

NATIONAL GEOGRAPHIC

WASHINGTON, D.C.

CONTENTS

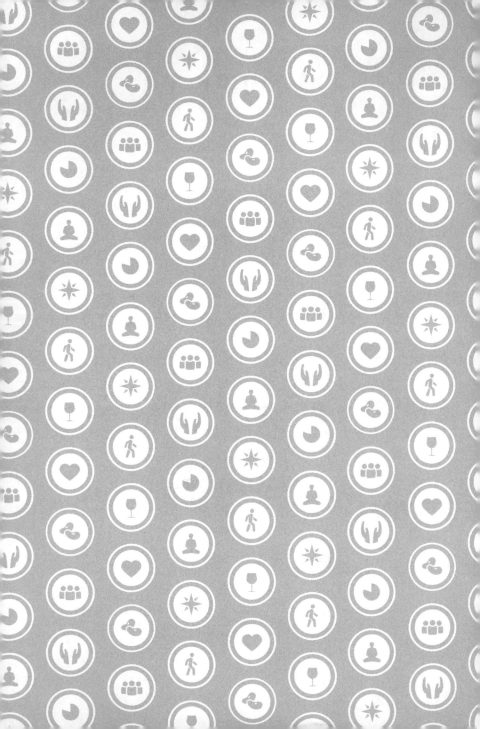

Introduction

I'm just going to say it. If you're overweight, suffering from diabetes, heart disease, or even several kinds of cancer, it's probably not your fault. Politicians like to shake their finger at us and tell us our health is up to us, that it's our "individual responsibility." I don't buy it.

Let's look at the numbers. Fifty years ago, Americans suffered one-third the current rate of obesity, one-seventh the rate of diabetes, and, by some measures, one-tenth the rate of dementia. Is that because we were more educated? Or were we somehow better people who took more responsibility for our own health?

No.

In 1960 there were only 100 McDonald's franchises in the United States; today there are 250,000 fast-food restaurants across the country. Before, you only found candy bars, chips, and soda in the grocery store. Now, more than 40 percent of all retail outlets, including pharmacies, tire repair shops, and plumbing supply stores require you to run a gauntlet of junk food to get to the cash register. Restaurant food portions—mostly meaty and cheesy—have grown to supersized proportions. And the processed food and beverage industry hires the sharpest minds on Madison Avenue and spends more than $10 billion a year to convince us to eat food that erodes our health.

To counter those health-eroding effects, we're then bamboozled into thinking that superfoods and powerboat nutra drinks are going to somehow make up for the junk. The vast majority of these are sugar-laden and actually accelerate weight gain. Add to this state of affairs the fact that we're genetically hardwired to crave fat, sugar, and salt. That's how 99 percent of the 25,000 generations of humans who came before us survived. For most of human history, we've lived in an environment of hardship and scarcity. Now we live in an environment of excess and ease. The processed food industry seizes on our hardwiring. They hire scientists to engineer junk food to achieve a highly addictive bliss point of savory and sweet. As former *New York Times* investigative journalist Michael Moss writes in his book *Hooked*, "The smoke from cigarettes takes 10 seconds to stir the brain, but a touch of sugar on the tongue will do so in a little more than a half second, or six hundred milliseconds, to be precise. That's nearly 20 times faster than cigarettes."

How are we supposed to make "responsible choices" in this food environment under a constant bombardment of psychological manipulation?

And it's not just food: We're also becoming more sedentary. Our grandparents expended more than five times as many calories engaging in non-exercise physical activity. They didn't have fancy gym memberships. Today, mechanical conveniences do most of our yard work, kitchen work, and household chores. (Anyone else have one of those robot vacuum cleaners?) We drive twice as many miles as we did in the 1970s, and fewer than 10 percent of our children walk to school, down from the high of 50 percent. Now, with online shopping, we don't even have to make the trip to the grocery store.

Finally, we're experiencing a crisis of loneliness. One in five Americans reports not having at least three friends "they can count on on a bad day." Loneliness can lead to depression, suicide, and poor health. Indeed, lonely people can expect to live eight years less than well-connected people do.

What can any of us do about this sad state of affairs?

About 20 years ago, working for National Geographic and with a grant from the National Institute on Aging, I started identifying and studying the longest-lived people, those who are in what we called the world's blue zones. These are people who have eluded heart disease, diabetes, dementia, and several types of cancer. My goal, in a sense, was to reverse engineer longevity. Since only about 20 percent of the average person's life span is dictated by genes, I reasoned that if I could find the common denominators among people who've achieved the health outcomes we want, I might distill some pretty good lessons for the rest of us to follow. I discovered nine powerful lessons—the Power 9® (page 21)—that underpin all five blue zones.

But the big insight was this: People who live a long time don't really know why they live a long time. They don't have heroic discipline, don't know something we don't, and they certainly have no more "individual responsibility" than we do. Their secret: They live in an environment where the healthy choice is not only the easy choice, but often the only choice. The cheapest, most accessible, and most delicious foods are whole, plant-based options. Every trip to the store, a friend's house, or to work occasions a walk. They have gardens out back. I've estimated that they're nudged into physical activity every 20 minutes or so. Loneliness is not an option. Every time they step out their front door, they bump into neighbors. They're expected to show up to church and to social gatherings; if they don't, there are friends and family pounding on their door. And they have vocabulary for purpose. They lead meaningful lives because they are clear on their values, passions, and talents—and they know where and how to put them to work.

For a dozen years, my company Blue Zones and I have helped more than 50 American cities reshape their environment for greater health and longevity. In the Beach Cities of California, we helped lower the obesity rate by 15 percent and lower smoking rates by more than 30 percent. In Fort Worth, Texas, we helped the city lower the collective body mass index, which occasioned a citywide health care savings of an estimated $250 million per year. We achieved this not by convincing a million people to buck up, find discipline, and get more responsible. We did it by shaping their surroundings to make the healthy choice easier. Where diet and exercise trends might doom them to failure, we set them up for success.

Unlike virtually every other health challenge, the Blue Zones Challenge focuses on setting up your environment to make healthy choices the easiest choices. By borrowing from the Power 9®, we can optimize the places we live, socialize, and work. Our homes can become mini blue zones, and along with our social network, we can expand the reach and improve the overall health of our immediate circle, including friends and family and even our greater community.

Individual change is hard—willpower runs out quickly. Most New Year's resolutions last just four to six weeks. The Blue Zones Challenge is designed to help you make over your own environment—in your kitchen, in your home, in your yard, in your office, and even in your social circle. Each aspect of the Blue Zones Challenge will help you create a lifestyle that supports longevity and a better quality of life.

This book is dedicated to you. In these pages, I've distilled my two decades of research in how to shape an environment to set you up for success. Just give me 30 days—one month of your life—to follow the recommendations on these pages. Take them seriously. I guarantee you that if you set up your surroundings the right way, a longer, better life awaits you. You can bet your life on it. I've bet mine on it.

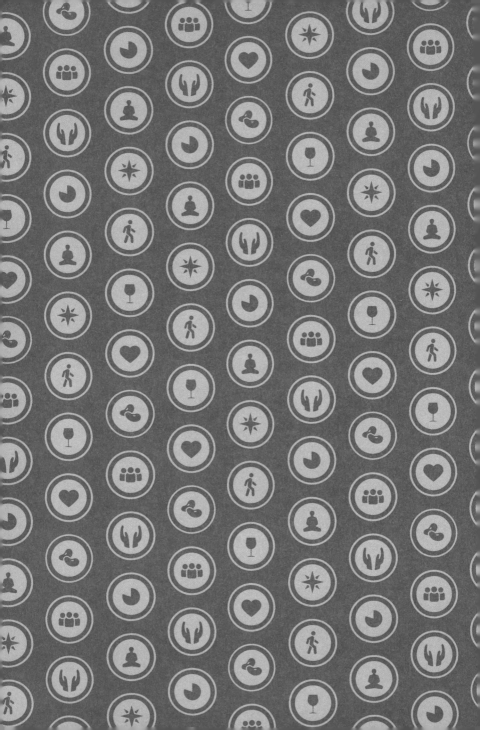

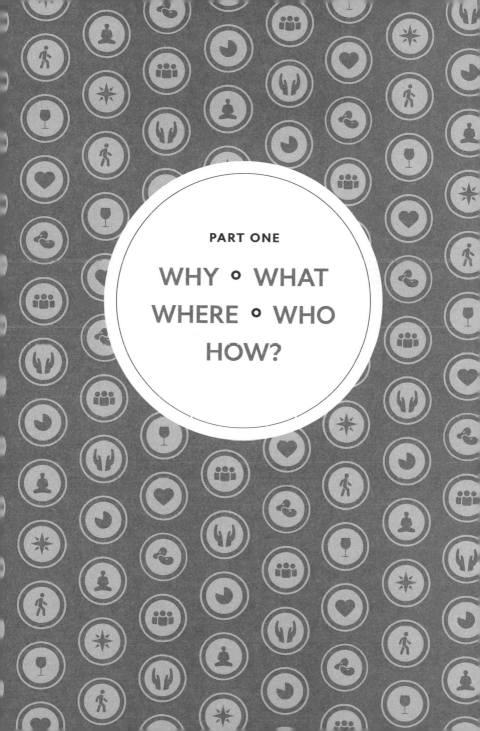

PART ONE

WHY ∘ WHAT
WHERE ∘ WHO
HOW?

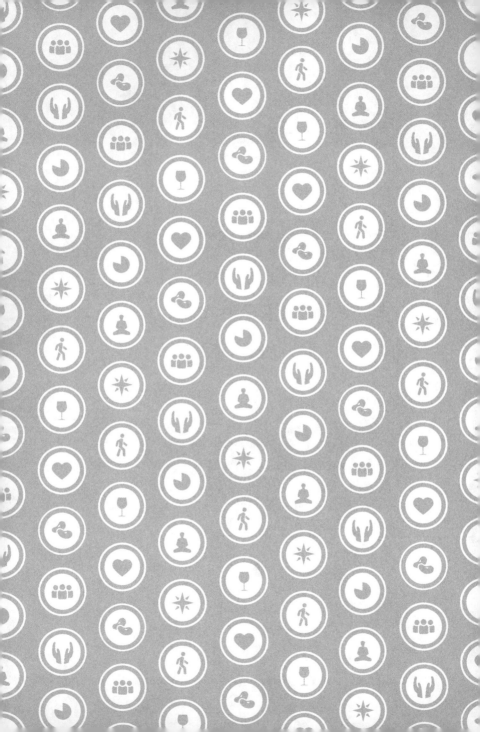

≋

Four Weeks to a Better, Happier, Less-Stressed Life

WELCOME TO THE BLUE ZONES CHALLENGE, four weeks to a better, happier, and less-stressed life. The Blue Zones Challenge is rooted in our groundbreaking research of the healthiest, longest-lived people on earth, but it's also informed by the latest scientific research and our work with communities all across the United States. It's not an elimination diet or a fitness plan. It's four weeks toward a better you. This is a new way to look at your health that will change your life for the better in nearly every way. Instead of focusing on behavior change and habit formation, we will help you improve the places and spaces in which you spend the most time (including your social circle!) to create the Blue Zones life you want.

WHY the Blue Zones Life?

You might come into the Blue Zones Challenge with goals like weight loss, but your health is oh so much more than a number on the scale. By following the challenge, you might lose weight, yes. But over time you will realize that weight loss is just one small benefit in a landslide of great outcomes. Consider the amazing long-term benefits that a Blue Zones life can help you with:

- Living a longer, better life
- Having more energy, feeling stronger, and having increased health
- Sleeping better and feeling rested every day
- Losing weight and learning to cook delicious meals at the same time
- Meeting new people and nurturing supportive relationships
- Discovering your purpose and putting it to work
- Being a change agent to help better your community

WHAT Makes the Blue Zones and the Power 9® Work?

The Blue Zones areas of the world share and benefit from a set of habits that we call the Power 9®, practices that—together—increase longevity, health, and happiness.

Our research has shown that these sets of behaviors and outlooks benefit people in the following ways:

- Longer, healthier life. Not just longevity for the sake of a number, but vitality. That means engagement with family, friends, and daily routines into your 90s and beyond.
- Lower rates of chronic diseases, such as Alzheimer's, cancer, depression, and dementia.
- Quality relationships. Part of the key to a life in alignment with Blue Zones habits is active engagement with community, friends, and family. These relationships work in a virtuous cycle of happiness and health: Spending quality time with others is not just enjoyable in the moment but it contributes to your overall health and that of your circle too!
- Adding life to your years, while adding years to your life. All of the Power 9® components help you to build a longer *and* better life.
- Increased satisfaction in life by having a purpose and being engaged in spiritual practice. Both of these are important to your quality of life and how you demonstrate your health and well-being outwardly.

WHERE Can We Find the Blue Zones in Action?

The original five blue zones can be found all over the planet, demonstrating how we can live healthy lives no matter what climate or country we are in. Those communities are Sardinia, Italy; the Nicoya Peninsula, Costa Rica; Okinawa, Japan; Loma Linda, California; and Ikaria, Greece. We started the Blue Zones Project® to use the wisdom of the original blue zones to tackle our current health crisis. It's now a solution in more than 50 communities around the United States, and has improved population health and reduced health care costs in a groundbreaking way.

In Blue Zones Project communities our teams of experts help cities set up ubiquitous nudges and defaults so the healthy choice is easy and natural. We help city governments choose and implement policies that favor fruits and vegetables over junk food and pedestrians over cars. We coach restaurants, grocery stores, schools, churches, and workplaces to nudge people to move naturally, socialize more, and eat healthier. Finally, we recruit 15 percent of the adult population to optimize their homes and social networks for better health. Where are some of the current projects?

- Albert Lea, Minnesota (the first location), where life span and community physical activity rocketed up and have stayed up for a full decade.
- Beach Cities, California, where childhood obesity

declined by 50 percent, smoking declined by 36 percent, and stress declined by 8 percent.

- Fort Worth, Texas, which transformed from one of the unhealthiest cities in the nation—the city's well-being rank rocketed to 31st from 185 out of 190 in the nation.
- Southwest Florida's Collier County, which went from 73rd in the country in well-being to first for four years in a row, and where heart disease deaths dropped by 8 percent to the lowest rate in the state.

These Blue Zones Project communities have shown that the benefits of blue zones can be built from the ground up.

WHO Practices the Blue Zones Power 9® and
HOW Has It Changed Them?

The Blue Zones Challenge is based on our research: the identification of the world's most extraordinary cultures whose health and longevity and happiness are outsized. People in blue zones didn't have to embark on a special program to transform their lives. Luckily for them, they live in places where moving naturally all day, eating healthily, and connecting with neighbors is the norm. In the spirit of those areas, we have brought environmental and cultural change to new places with the Blue Zones Project. We help change health and well-being by showing communities how they can remake their environments, social groups, and individual lifestyles.

When creating the Blue Zones Challenge, we looked to the original blue zones, each Blue Zones Project community, and the latest developments in the science of well-being. We use research-backed and evidence-based interventions in all our work.

Reverse Engineering Longevity

The life expectancy of an American born today averages 78.2 years. But in 2021, more than 70,000 Americans have reached their 100th birthday. What are they doing that the average American isn't?

To answer the question, I teamed up with National Geographic to find the world's longest-lived people and study them. We knew most of the answer lay within their lifestyle and environment—the Danish Twin Study established that only about 20 percent of the length of an average person's life is determined by genes. Then I gathered a team of scientists and demographers to find pockets of people around the world with the highest life expectancy, or with the highest proportions of people who reach age 100.

We found five places that met our criteria:

- The Barbagia region of Sardinia—mountainous highlands of inner Sardinia with the world's highest concentration of male centenarians.

- Ikaria, Greece—Aegean island with one of the world's lowest rates of middle-age mortality and the lowest rates of dementia.
- Nicoya Peninsula, Costa Rica—region with the world's lowest rates of middle-age mortality, and the second highest concentration of male centenarians.
- Loma Linda, California—where there's a high concentration of Seventh-day Adventists, who on average live 10 years longer than their North American counterparts.
- Okinawa, Japan—where females over 70 are the longest-lived population in the world.

I then assembled a team of medical researchers, anthropologists, demographers, and epidemiologists to search for evidence-based common denominators among all the places. We found nine—what ultimately led to the Blue Zones Power 9®.

Blue Zones Power 9®

Lifestyle Habits of the World's Healthiest, Longest-Lived People

1. Move Naturally

The world's longest-lived people don't pump iron, run marathons, or join gyms. Instead, they live in environments that constantly nudge them into moving without thinking about it. They grow gardens and don't have mechanical conveniences for house and yard work.

2. Purpose

The Okinawans call it *ikigai* and the Nicoyans call it *plan de vida;* for both it translates to "why I wake up in the morning." Knowing your sense of purpose is worth up to seven years of extra life expectancy.

3. Downshift

Even people in the Blue Zones experience stress. Stress leads to chronic inflammation, associated with every major age-related disease. What the world's longest-lived people have that we don't are routines to shed that stress. Okinawans take a few moments each day to remember their ancestors, Adventists pray, Ikarians take a nap, and Sardinians do happy hour.

4. 80 Percent Rule

Hara hachi bu, the Okinawan, 2,500-year-old Confucian mantra said before meals, reminds them to stop eating when their stomachs are 80 percent full. The 20 percent gap between not being hungry and feeling full could be the difference between losing weight and gaining it. People in the blue zones eat their smallest meal in the late afternoon or early evening and then they don't eat any more for the rest of the day.

5. Plant Slant

Beans, including fava, black, soy, and lentils, are the cornerstone of most centenarian diets. Meat—mostly pork—is eaten on average only five times per month. Serving sizes are three to four ounces, about the size of a deck of cards.

6. Wine @ 5

People in all blue zones (except Adventists) drink alcohol moderately and regularly. Moderate drinkers outlive nondrinkers. The trick is to drink one to two glasses per day (preferably Sardinian Cannonau wine), with friends and/or with food. And no, you can't save up all week and have 14 drinks on Saturday.

7. Belong

All but five of the 263 centenarians we interviewed belonged to some faith-based community. Denomination doesn't seem to matter. Research shows that attending faith-based services four times per month will add four to 14 years of life expectancy.

8. Loved Ones First

Successful centenarians in the blue zones put their families first. This means keeping aging parents and grandparents nearby or in the home. (It lowers disease and mortality rates of children in the home too.) They commit to a life partner (which can add up to three years of life expectancy) and invest in their children with time and love (and they'll be more likely to care for you when the time comes).

9. Right Tribe

The world's longest-lived people chose—or were born into—social circles that support healthy behaviors. For example, Okinawans created *moais*—groups of five friends that committed to each other for life. Research from the Framingham Studies shows that smoking, obesity, happiness, and even loneliness are contagious. So the social networks of long-lived people have favorably shaped their health behaviors.

To make it to age 100, you have to have won the genetic lottery. But most of us have the capacity to make it well into our early 90s and largely without chronic disease. As the Adventists demonstrate, the average person's life expectancy could increase by 10 to 12 years by adopting a Blue Zones lifestyle.

POWER 9®

Copyright Blue Zones, LLC

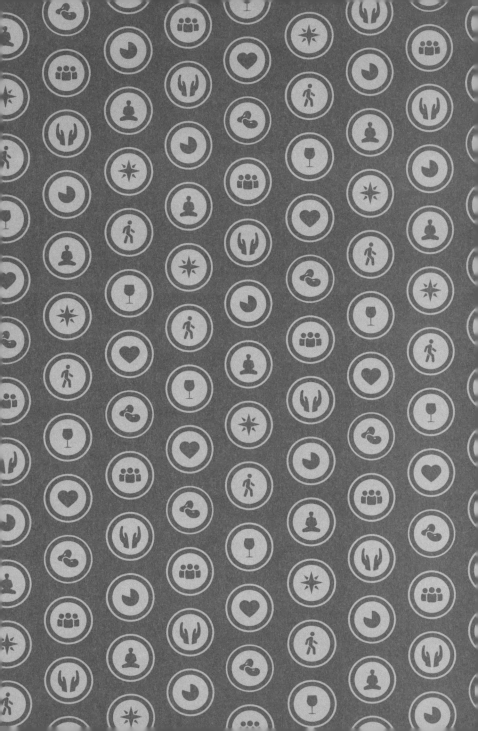

PART TWO

WELCOME TO
THE BLUE ZONES
OF THE WORLD

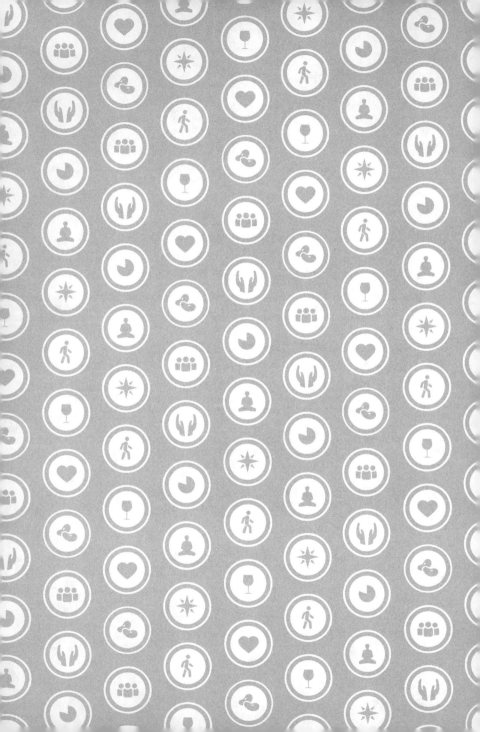

≈

Home to the World's Most Extraordinary Cultures

THE FOUNDATION FOR THE BLUE ZONES CHALLENGE LIVES IN THE WORLD'S BLUE ZONES. During my 40 or so trips to the blue zones of the world, I spent time just sitting with 100-year-olds and listening to their stories and paying attention to their lives. I watched them prepare their meals and ate what they had been eating their whole lives. Wherever I found long-lived populations, I found similar habits and practices. Their houses and dishes may have looked and sounded different, but their lifestyles were remarkably similar.

Sardinia, Italy
. . . .
Home to the World's Longest-Living Men

A cluster of villages in a kidney-shaped region on this island makes up the first blue zones region we ever identified. In 2004, our research team set off to investigate a rare genetic quirk carried by its inhabitants. The M26 marker is linked to exceptional longevity, and because of the geographic isolation of the residents in this area of Sardinia, their genes have remained mostly undiluted. The result: nearly 10 times more centenarians per capita than in the United States.

But even more important, residents of this area are also culturally isolated, and they have kept to a very traditional, healthy lifestyle. Sardinians still grow, harvest, catch, and raise the food they eat. They remain close with friends and family throughout their lives. They laugh and drink wine together.

Lessons From Sardinia

Eat a plant-based diet accented with meat.
The classic Sardinian diet consists of whole-grain bread, beans, garden vegetables, fruits, and, in some parts of the island, mastic oil (an oil from a tree related to the pistachio tree, which has antibacterial properties). Sardinians also traditionally eat pecorino cheese made from grass-fed sheep, whose cheese is high in omega-3

fatty acids. Goat's milk is the dairy of choice, and meat is largely reserved for Sundays and special occasions.

Put family first.

Sardinia's strong family values help ensure that every member of the family is cared for. People who live in strong, healthy families suffer lower rates of depression, suicide, and stress.

Celebrate elders.

Grandparents can provide love, childcare, financial help, wisdom, and the expectation/motivation to continue traditions and push children to succeed in their lives. This may all add up to healthier, better-adjusted, and longer-lived children. It may give the overall population a life expectancy bump.

Take a walk.

Walking five miles or more a day, as Sardinian shepherds do, provides all the cardiovascular benefits you might expect, and also has a positive effect on muscle and bone metabolism without the joint pounding of running marathons or triathlons.

Drink a glass or two of red wine daily.

Sardinians drink wine moderately. Cannonau wine has two or three times the level of artery-scrubbing flavonoids as other wines. Moderate wine consumption may help explain the lower levels of stress among men.

Laugh with friends.
Men in this blue zones region are famous for their sardonic sense of humor. They gather in the street each afternoon to laugh with and at each other. Laughter reduces stress, which can lower one's risk of cardiovascular disease.

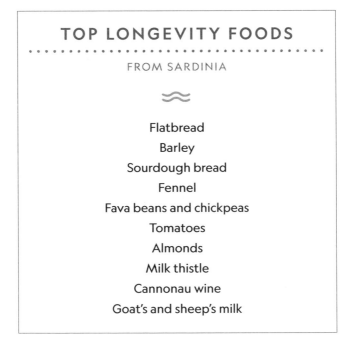

TOP LONGEVITY FOODS

FROM SARDINIA

Flatbread
Barley
Sourdough bread
Fennel
Fava beans and chickpeas
Tomatoes
Almonds
Milk thistle
Cannonau wine
Goat's and sheep's milk

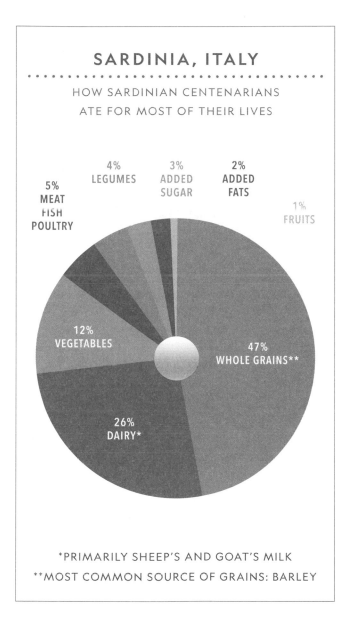

SARDINIA, ITALY

HOW SARDINIAN CENTENARIANS
ATE FOR MOST OF THEIR LIVES

4%
LEGUMES

3%
ADDED
SUGAR

2%
ADDED
FATS

5%
MEAT
FISH
POULTRY

1%
FRUITS

12%
VEGETABLES

47%
WHOLE GRAINS**

26%
DAIRY*

*PRIMARILY SHEEP'S AND GOAT'S MILK
**MOST COMMON SOURCE OF GRAINS: BARLEY

Ikaria, Greece
The Island Where People Forget to Die

This tiny island's long history has been as rocky as its topography. The outcropping in the Aegean Sea has been the target of invasions by Persians, Romans, and Turks, forcing its residents inland from the coasts. The result: An isolated culture rich in tradition, family values, and longevity.

Today, older Ikarians are almost entirely free of dementia and some of the chronic diseases that plague Americans; one in three makes it to their 90s. A combination of factors explain it, including geography, culture, diet, lifestyle, and outlook. They enjoy strong red wine, late-night domino games, and a relaxed pace of life that ignores clocks. Clean air, warm breezes, and rugged terrain draw them outdoors into an active lifestyle.

Ikarians have woven the recipe for longevity into their culture and lifestyle. Follow these common practices to cultivate your own centenarian lifestyle.

Lessons From Ikaria

Mimic mountain living.

The longest-lived Ikarians tend to be poor people living in the island's highlands. They exercise mindlessly by just gardening, walking to their neighbor's house, or doing their own yard work. The lesson to us: Engineer more mindless movement into our lives.

Eat a Mediterranean-style diet.

Ikarians eat a variation of the Mediterranean diet, with lots of fruits and vegetables, whole grains, beans, potatoes, and olive oil. Try cooking with olive oil, which contains cholesterol-lowering monounsaturated fats.

Stock up on herbs.

People in Ikaria enjoy drinking herbal teas with family and friends, and scientists have found that those teas pack an antioxidant punch. Wild rosemary, sage, and oregano teas also act as a diuretic, which can keep blood pressure in check by ridding the body of excess sodium and water.

Nap.

Take a cue from Ikarians and take a midafternoon break. People who nap regularly have up to a 35 percent lower chance of dying from heart disease. It may be because napping lowers stress hormones or rests the heart.

Fast occasionally.

Ikarians have traditionally been fierce Greek Orthodox Christians. Their religious calendar calls for fasting almost half the year. Caloric restriction—a type of fasting that cuts about 30 percent of the calories out of a normal diet—is the only scientifically proven way to slow the aging process in mammals.

Make family and friends a priority.
Ikarians foster social connections, which have been shown to benefit overall health and longevity. So get out there and make some plans.

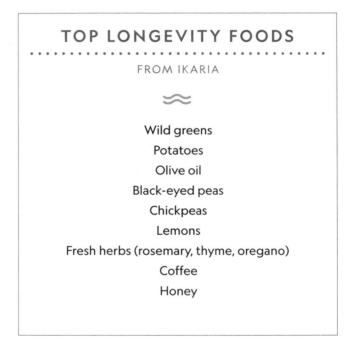

TOP LONGEVITY FOODS

FROM IKARIA

Wild greens
Potatoes
Olive oil
Black-eyed peas
Chickpeas
Lemons
Fresh herbs (rosemary, thyme, oregano)
Coffee
Honey

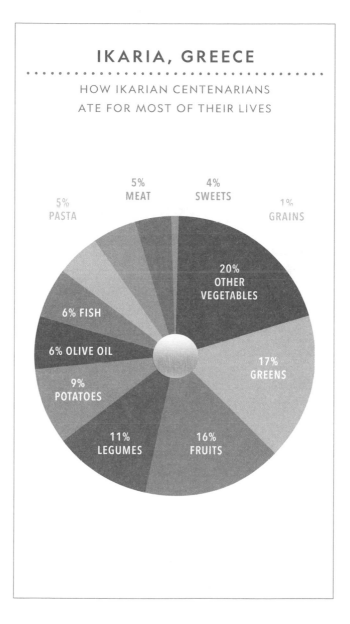

IKARIA, GREECE

· ·

HOW IKARIAN CENTENARIANS
ATE FOR MOST OF THEIR LIVES

5%
PASTA

5%
MEAT

4%
SWEETS

1%
GRAINS

20%
OTHER
VEGETABLES

6% FISH

6% OLIVE OIL

17%
GREENS

9%
POTATOES

11%
LEGUMES

16%
FRUITS

Loma Linda, California, U.S.A.
. . . .
A Group of Americans Living 10 Years Longer

The Seventh-day Adventist Church in this sunny pocket of Southern California was founded in the 1840s. The church flourished through the 20th century—and so did its members, who view health as central to their faith.

Today, a community of about 9,000 Adventists in the Loma Linda area are the core of America's blue zones region. They live as much as a decade longer than the rest of us, and much of their longevity can be attributed to vegetarianism and regular exercise. Plus, Adventists don't smoke or drink alcohol.

How can you live like the American longevity all-stars? Try these tactics practiced in Loma Linda to live measurably longer.

Lessons From Loma Linda

Find a sanctuary in time.
A weekly break from the rigors of daily life, the 24-hour Sabbath provides a time to focus on family, God, camaraderie, and nature. Adventists claim this relieves their stress, strengthens social networks, and provides consistent exercise.

Maintain a healthy body mass index (BMI).

Adventists have healthier BMIs (meaning they have a more appropriate weight for their height) than the average American, and lacto-ovo vegetarian Adventists have even healthier BMIs than nonvegetarians. Studies correlate excess weight with higher risk of heart attack, stroke, high blood pressure, diabetes, arthritis, and several cancers.

Get regular, moderate exercise.

The Adventist Health Survey (AHS) shows that you don't need to be a marathoner to maximize your life expectancy. Getting regular, low-intensity exercise like daily walks appears to help reduce your chance of having heart disease and certain cancers.

Spend time with like-minded friends.

Adventists tend to spend time with lots of other Adventists. They find well-being by sharing one another's values and supporting one another's habits.

Snack on nuts.

Adventists who consume nuts at least five times a week have about half the risk of heart disease and live about two years longer than those who don't. At least four major studies have confirmed that eating nuts has a positive impact on health and life expectancy.

Give something back.

Like many faiths, the Seventh-day Adventist Church encourages and provides opportunities for its members to volunteer. Often the centenarians we spoke with stay active, find sense of purpose, and stave off depression by focusing on helping others.

Avoid meat.

Many Adventists follow a vegetarian or vegan diet. The AHS shows that consuming fruits and vegetables and whole grains seems to be protective against a wide variety of cancers. The longest-lived Adventists are vegetarian or pescatarian.

Eat an early, light dinner.

"Eat breakfast like a king, lunch like a prince, and dinner like a pauper," American nutritionist Adelle Davis is said to have recommended—an attitude also reflected in Adventist practices. A light dinner early in the evening avoids flooding the body with calories during the inactive parts of the day. It also seems to promote better sleep and a lower BMI.

Put more plants in your diet.

In support of a biblical diet of grains, fruits, nuts, and vegetables, Adventists cite Genesis 1:29: "And God said, Behold, I have given you every herb bearing seed, which is upon the face of all the earth, and every tree, in which is the fruit of a tree yielding seed; to you it shall be for meat." The Adventists encourage a "well-balanced diet" including nuts, fruits, and legumes, low in sugar, salt, and refined grains. Studies have shown that nonsmoking Adventists who ate two or more servings of fruit per day had about 70 percent fewer lung cancers than nonsmokers who ate fruit just once or twice a week. Adventists who ate legumes such as peas and beans three times a week had a 30 to 40 percent reduction in colon cancer.

Adventist women who consumed tomatoes at least three or four times a week reduced their chance of getting ovarian cancer by 70 percent over those who ate tomatoes less often. Eating a lot of tomatoes also seemed to have an effect on reducing prostate cancer for men. A new study has found that adherents to this way of life have the nation's lowest rates of heart disease and diabetes and very low rates of obesity.

Drink plenty of water.

The AHS suggests that men who drank five or six daily glasses of water had a substantial reduction in the risk of a fatal heart attack—60 to 70 percent—compared to those who drank considerably less.

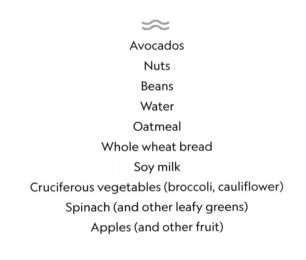

TOP LONGEVITY FOODS

FROM LOMA LINDA

Avocados

Nuts

Beans

Water

Oatmeal

Whole wheat bread

Soy milk

Cruciferous vegetables (broccoli, cauliflower)

Spinach (and other leafy greens)

Apples (and other fruit)

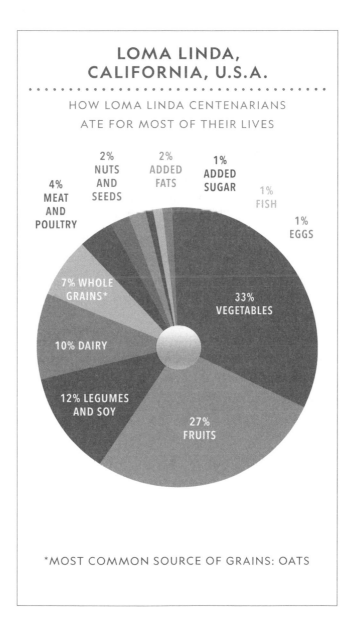

LOMA LINDA, CALIFORNIA, U.S.A.

HOW LOMA LINDA CENTENARIANS
ATE FOR MOST OF THEIR LIVES

2%
NUTS
AND
SEEDS

2%
ADDED
FATS

1%
ADDED
SUGAR

1%
FISH

4%
MEAT
AND
POULTRY

1%
EGGS

7% WHOLE
GRAINS*

33%
VEGETABLES

10% DAIRY

12% LEGUMES
AND SOY

27%
FRUITS

*MOST COMMON SOURCE OF GRAINS: OATS

Okinawa, Japan
· ·
Secrets of the World's Longest-Living Women

The islands at the southern end of Japan, once called the land of immortals, have historically been known for longevity. Older Okinawans have traditionally had less cancer, heart disease, and dementia than Americans, and women there live longer than any other women on the planet.

Perhaps their greatest secret is a strong dedication to friends and family. They maintain a powerful social network called a *moai*, a lifelong circle of friends that supports people well into old age. Okinawans also have a strong sense of purpose in life, a driving force that the Japanese call *ikigai*.

Despite years of hardship, older generations of Okinawans have established a lifestyle and environment in which to live long, healthy lives. Follow these common centenarian practices to promote your own longevity.

Lessons From Okinawa

Embrace an *ikigai*.
Older Okinawans can readily articulate the reason they get up in the morning. Their purpose-imbued lives give them clear roles of responsibility and feelings of being needed well into their 100s.

Rely on a plant-based diet.

Older Okinawans have eaten a plant-based diet most of their lives. Their meals of stir-fried vegetables, sweet potatoes, and tofu are high in nutrients and low in calories. Goya, or bitter melon, with its antioxidants and compounds that lower blood sugar, is of particular interest. While centenarian Okinawans do eat some pork, it is traditionally reserved only for infrequent ceremonial occasions and taken only in small amounts.

Get gardening.

Almost all Okinawan centenarians grow or once grew a garden. It's a source of daily physical activity that exercises the body with a wide range of motion and helps reduce stress. It's also a near-constant source of fresh vegetables.

Eat more soy.

The Okinawan diet is rich in foods made with soy, such as tofu and miso soup. Flavonoids in tofu may help protect the heart and guard against breast cancer. Fermented soy foods contribute to a healthy intestinal ecology and offer even better nutritional benefits.

Maintain a *moai*.

The Okinawan tradition of forming a *moai* provides secure social networks. These safety nets lend financial and emotional support in times of need and give all of their members the stress-shedding security of knowing that there is always someone there for them.

Enjoy the sunshine.
Vitamin D, produced by the body when it's exposed on a regular basis to sunlight, promotes stronger bones and healthier bodies. Spending time outside each day allows even senior Okinawans to have optimal vitamin D levels year-round.

Stay active.
Older Okinawans are active walkers and gardeners. The Okinawan household has very little furniture; residents take meals and relax sitting on tatami mats on the floor. The fact that old people get up and down off the floor several dozen times daily builds lower body strength and balance, which help protect against dangerous falls.

Plant a medical garden.
Mugwort, ginger, and turmeric are all staples of an Okinawan garden, and all have proven medicinal qualities. By consuming these every day, Okinawans may be protecting themselves against illness.

Have an attitude.
A hardship-tempered attitude has endowed Okinawans with an affable smugness. They're able to let difficult early years remain in the past while they enjoy today's

simple pleasures. They've learned to be likable and to keep younger people in their company well into their old age.

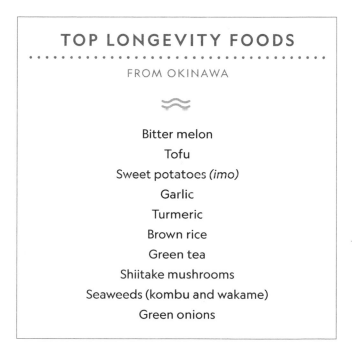

TOP LONGEVITY FOODS

FROM OKINAWA

Bitter melon
Tofu
Sweet potatoes *(imo)*
Garlic
Turmeric
Brown rice
Green tea
Shiitake mushrooms
Seaweeds (kombu and wakame)
Green onions

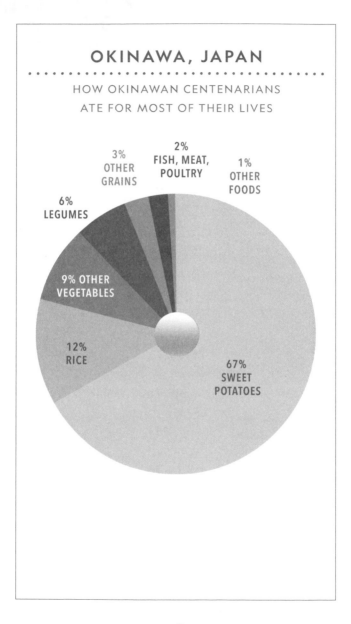

OKINAWA, JAPAN

HOW OKINAWAN CENTENARIANS
ATE FOR MOST OF THEIR LIVES

3%
OTHER
GRAINS

2%
FISH, MEAT,
POULTRY

1%
OTHER
FOODS

6%
LEGUMES

9% OTHER
VEGETABLES

12%
RICE

67%
SWEET
POTATOES

THE RISE (AND LATER FALL)
OF A GREAT LONGEVITY DIET

Okinawa is sort of a Japanese Hawaii—an exotic, laid-back group of islands with warm weather, palm trees, and sugar-sand beaches. For almost a thousand years, this Pacific archipelago has maintained a reputation for nurturing extreme longevity. Okinawans over the age of 65 enjoy the world's highest life expectancy: Men are expected to live to about 84, while women are expected to live to almost age 90. They suffer only a fraction of the diseases that kill Americans: one-fifth the rate of cardiovascular disease, one-fifth the rate of breast and prostate cancer, and less than half the rate of dementia seen among similarly aged Americans.

At the time of our study and research on the island over the last 20 years, most of the Okinawans age 100 or more who were alive were born between 1903 and 1914. During the first third of their lives, roughly before 1940, the vast majority of the calories they consumed—more than 60 percent—came from one food: the *imo,* or Okinawan sweet potato. A purple or yellow variety related to our orange sweet potato, the *imo* came to the islands from the Americas about 400 years ago and took well to Okinawan soils. This sweet potato—high in flavonoids, vitamin C, fiber, carotenoids, and slow-burning carbohydrates—is one of the healthiest foods on the planet.

The traditional Okinawan diet was about 80 percent carbohydrates. Before 1940 Okinawans also consumed fish at least three times per week together with seven servings of vegetables and maybe one or two servings of grains per day. They also ate two servings of flavonoid-rich soy, usually in the form of tofu. They didn't eat much fruit; they enjoyed a few eggs a week. Dairy and meat represented only about 3 percent of their calories. On special occasions, usually during the Lunar New Year, people butchered the family pig and feasted on pork.

The meat in their diet gave me pause. When I first struck off on my blue zones research in 2000, I was absolutely convinced that I'd find that a vegan diet yielded the greatest health and life expectancy. So when I discovered that older Okinawans not only ate pork but loved it, I thought their example must be an outlier—that they were living long despite pork. Pork is high in saturated fat, which, when consumed in excess, often leads to heart disease. But again, we learned a few lessons. Okinawans stewed the pork for days, cooking out and skimming off the fat. What they ate, in the end, was the high-protein collagen.

Fast Food Invasion

As healthful as they were, some of these Okinawan food traditions foundered mid-century. Following World War II, Western influences—and economic prosperity—crept into traditional life and food habits changed. Okinawans doubled their rice consumption, and bread, virtually unknown before, also slid in. Milk consumption increased; meat, eggs, and poultry consumption increased more than sevenfold. Between 1949 and 1972 Okinawans' daily nutritional intake increased by 400 calories. They were consuming more than 200 calories per day more than they needed—like Americans. Cancers of the lung, breast, and colon almost doubled.

Yet older Okinawans, whose diets had solidified before that time period, are still the world's longest-lived people.

Nicoya, Costa Rica
A Latin American Blue Zones Region

This Central American nation isn't that far from the U.S. geographically, but it is way ahead of us in longevity. Costa Rica is economically secure and has excellent health care. But other factors are at play, especially in Nicoya, an 80-mile peninsula just south of the Nicaraguan border.

One is the *plan de vida*, or "reason to live," which propels a positive outlook among elders and helps keep them active. Another is a focus on family and a special ability to listen and laugh. Nicoyan centenarians frequently visit with neighbors, and they tend to live with family and children or grandchildren who provide support, as well as a sense of purpose.

This information has been translated into lessons that can be implemented into your everyday life.

Lessons From Nicoya

Have a *plan de vida*.

Successful centenarians have a strong sense of purpose. They feel needed and want to contribute to a greater good.

Drink hard water.

Nicoyan water has the country's highest calcium content, perhaps explaining the lower rates of heart disease, as well as stronger bones and fewer hip fractures.

Keep a focus on family.

Nicoyan centenarians tend to live with their families, and children or grandchildren provide support and a sense of purpose and belonging.

Eat a light dinner.

Eating fewer calories appears to be one of the surest ways to add years to your life. Nicoyans eat a light dinner early in the evening. For most of their lives, Nicoyan centenarians ate a traditional Mesoamerican diet highlighted by the "three sisters" of agriculture: squash, corn, and beans.

Maintain social networks.

Nicoyan centenarians get frequent visits from neighbors. They know how to listen, laugh, and appreciate what they have.

Keep hard at work.

Centenarians seem to have enjoyed physical work of all their lives. They find joy in everyday physical chores, including gardening, maintaining their land, cooking, and caring for their grandchildren.

Get some sensible sun.

Nicoyans regularly take in the sunshine, which helps their bodies produce vitamin D for strong bones and healthy body function. Vitamin D deficiency is associated with a host of problems, such as osteoporosis and heart disease, but regular "smart" sun exposure (about 15 minutes on the legs and arms) can help supplement your diet and make sure you're getting enough of this vital nutrient.

Embrace a common history.

Modern Nicoyans' roots to the indigenous Chorotega and their traditions have enabled them to remain relatively free of stress. Their traditional diet of fortified maize and beans may be the best nutritional combination for longevity the world has ever known.

TOP LONGEVITY FOODS

FROM NICOYA

Maize nixtamal
(cornmeal soaked in lime and water)
Squash
Papayas
Yams
Black beans
Bananas
Peach palms
Mini sweet peppers
Cilantro and culantro coyote
Yuca

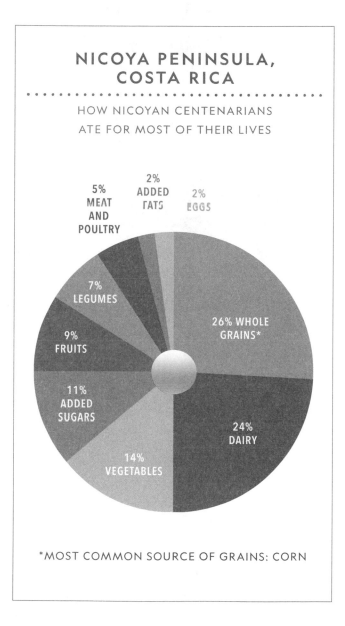

NICOYA PENINSULA, COSTA RICA

HOW NICOYAN CENTENARIANS ATE FOR MOST OF THEIR LIVES

5% MEAT AND POULTRY

2% ADDED FATS

2% EGGS

7% LEGUMES

9% FRUITS

11% ADDED SUGARS

14% VEGETABLES

24% DAIRY

26% WHOLE GRAINS*

*MOST COMMON SOURCE OF GRAINS: CORN

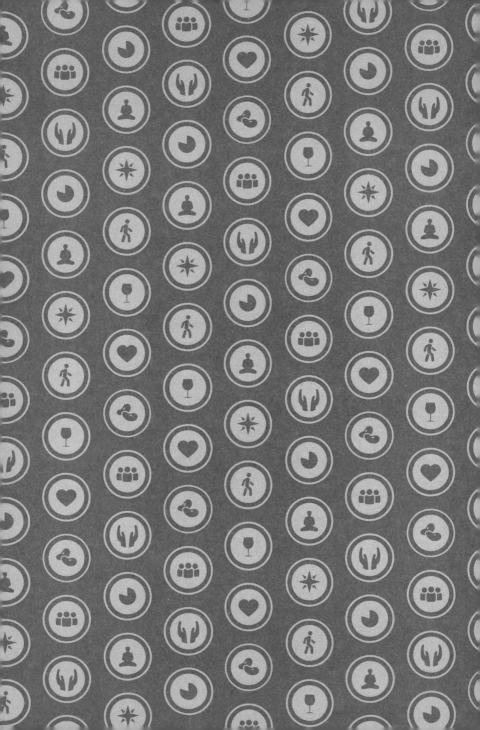

PART THREE

START THE CHALLENGE

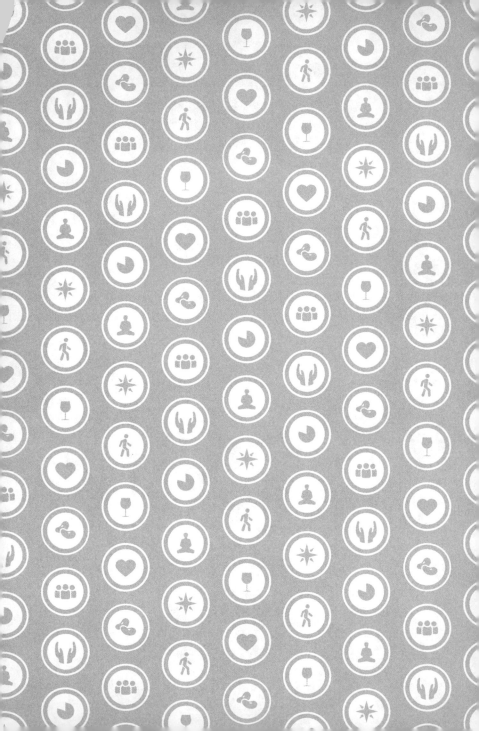

≋

The Blue Zones Life Challenge

How to Set Up Your Life—and Place and Spaces—to Create the Blue Zones Life You Want

B LUE ZONES CENTENARIANS AND NONAGENARIANS live in environments, villages, and towns that set them up for success. During the next four weeks, we are going to help you set up your life for success.

For the first week, you will set up your home, surroundings, and even your social life to support better health. You'll also take time this week to measure where you are starting from with some Blue Zones diagnostic tools. "You can't manage it if you can't measure it" holds true for most pursuits, including health and longevity. Tracking your progress also kick-starts the process of paying attention to what you do and eat as you set up your life, home, and surroundings to live the Blue Zones life.

Then we are going to ask you to spend the next three weeks keeping daily checklists that are all in the service of setting up your life for better health so you effortlessly make better decisions. We'll show you how to design your home, your social life, and your schedule so the healthy choice is the easy choice.

The goal of this challenge is to:

1. Give you the secrets of the world's longest-lived people and make sure you're convinced. For this, we're going to ask you to do a little reading and perhaps watch a video or two.

2. Show you how to set up your surroundings so that the Blue Zones healthy choice is the easy choice. For instance, you make more than 200 food decisions every day. Only 10 percent or so are conscious. We want your unconscious decisions to be healthy. We're also going to show you how to set up nudges and defaults so you move more every day, eat less, socialize more, and live out your purpose. Every one of these characteristics drives Blue Zones longevity and is supported by strong academic evidence.

3. Upgrade your social network—the most profound, measurable, and long-lasting thing you can do is build a social circle around yourself that supports healthy eating, activity, and emotional well-being. This may take more than a little effort on your part but the payoff is enormous and lasting.

4. Get you to eat a whole, plant-based, and lower-sugar (i.e., Blue Zones) diet for a month. Research from Harvard and an international group of scientists

shows overwhelmingly that the closer you can come to eating this way, the less likely you will be to develop heart disease, diabetes, dementia, and several types of cancer. This will probably be the hardest part of the next month. But we promise you: If you learn a handful of plant-based recipes that you like, and build a social network around eating healthily, it will be easy to do for the rest of your life. We also believe you will see immediate results this month: You'll shed weight, feel better, have clearer skin, gain more energy, and sleep better. You might even have better sex (see page 104 for more information on plant-based diets).

Week One
Set Up for Success

Winston Churchill famously said, "Shape your surroundings and they will shape you." Your first week of the Blue Zones Challenge is to begin to reshape your surroundings for the better. You will look at your current situation to get a baseline measurement and also prepare your schedule, home, and support system for the rest of the month.

Centenarians in blue zones regions didn't plan to live a long time, track what they ate, or do any health challenges. So why are we asking you to do some of these things? For most of us in the United States, our homes, neighborhoods, schools, workplaces, streets, and towns are set up to support convenience—including fast, calorie-rich, and nutrient-poor foods and a life spent sitting (at your desk, in your car, on your couch)—rather than well-being. In blue zones regions, the healthy choice is the default choice—people move naturally all day, have strong social support systems, and eat healthy foods most of the time because their environments nudge them to these behaviors all day, every day.

To live the Blue Zones life, we have to reengineer our current surroundings to replicate some of the ancient, time-honored practices we know support health and longevity. Unlike other plans and challenges, the Blue Zones lifestyle is sustainable. Although we encourage you to pay attention and come back often to the Blue Zones tools to see how you're doing, setting up your home, social circle, and schedule will make living the Blue Zones life a joy and not a chore.

Although we call this "week one," this process can take you up to 10 days. Take the time you need, as this setup week will make the rest of the month easier.

Step 1: Test yourself.

1. Take the **True Vitality Test** (page 66) and record your results.
2. Take the **True Happiness Test** (page 71) and record your results.

3. Take the **Purpose Checkup** (page 76) and write
   your **Purpose Statement** (page 84; this exercise
   can take multiple days). Hang your Purpose
   Statement by your desk or in a place you will see
   it every day.

True Vitality Test results: _____

True Happiness Test results: _____

Purpose Checkup results: _____

Step 2: Find a Blue Zones buddy or create a *moai* (either a walking or a potluck one).

See page 90 for tips and tricks to set up your very own *moai*.

Step 3: Set up your home for better health by design.

In the Kitchen:

- Post the list of **Four Always, Four to Avoid** foods
  in your kitchen (page 102).
- Post the **Blue Zones Food Guidelines** in your
  kitchen (page 112).
- Stock up on Always foods and other Blue Zones
  staples.
- Remove the Avoid foods from your house (or hide
  them on a top shelf or in a drawer for other family
  members, if needed).

In the Rest of Your Home:

- Put your walking or running shoes out where you can see them. (If you don't have running shoes or a bike, consider investing in them.)
- Set up a place or corner of your home with pillows where you can sit, read, or do work on the ground (page 114).
- Buy a scale or put yours in your bathroom or bedroom in a convenient place where you'll be encouraged to check your weight (page 115).
- Record your starting weight.

Starting Weight: _____

Optional: If you can, record your starting blood pressure, heart rate, blood sugar, and cholesterol.

Starting Blood Pressure: _____
Starting Heart Rate: _____
Starting Blood Sugar: _____
Starting Cholesterol: _____

Step 4: Wear a blue bracelet or other blue jewelry (a ring, watch, etc.) as a reminder of *hara hachi bu*.

Remind yourself of the Okinawan blessing said before meals to help you eat only until you're 80 percent full (see page 240 to learn about *hara hachi bu*).

Optional Tasks This Week:

- Buy an electric pressure cooker (either generic or name brand like Instant Pot).

- Buy microwave-safe food storage containers (I like Pyrex) or recycle glass pasta sauce jars, pickle jars, and other glass bottles for leftovers and meal prep.

- Do a mapping exercise to identify walking and biking routes in your neighborhood: Draw a map of your neighborhood with the streets, parks, cafés, homes of people you know, landmark buildings, places to go, and anything else important that you might walk or bike to. You can use Google Maps to help you identify places you might not have explored in your town or city.

Test Yourself

To start, see where you currently stand with the Blue Zones tests and the Purpose Checkup. Are you as happy as you'd like to be? How is your projected life expectancy compared to where it could be? And is your purpose defined? Things measured are the things that are managed. Just knowing where you start will help you see the real benefits and find ongoing momentum. Writing your Purpose Statement could take the longest and might even require a couple of days for you to perfect. Record your results from your tests and hang up your Purpose Statement where you will see it every day. Measuring your progress is a fantastic motivator to keep going for as long as it takes to make the changes permanent and your life better.

True Vitality Test

Created in collaboration with the University of Minnesota School of Public Health and based on more than 250 studies, the Blue Zones True Vitality Test calculates your healthy life expectancy and gives you a baseline read on how you're doing. You'll also get personalized recommendations for getting the most good years out of life.

Do this at the beginning and the end of the four-week challenge. You can't manage what you don't measure.

Results include your:
- Biological age
- Overall life expectancy
- Healthy life expectancy
- Years you're gaining/losing because of your habits
- Up to 12 customized recommendations to help you live longer

Please note: You do have to give your email in order to take the test online and receive your personalized recommendations. We keep your results and submissions private.

To receive your personalized recommendations, you will need to take the test online at apps.bluezones.com/ en/vitality. The entire test takes three to four minutes.

Here are the questions you will be asked:

Background

1. What year were you born?
2. Sex: male or female?
3. Where do you live?
4. What is your ethnicity?
5. What is your height?
6. What is your weight?
7. What was your weight two years ago?
8. What is your annual household income from all sources?
9. What was the last year of school you completed?
10. Have you smoked tobacco products in the last five years?
11. If you smoke now, how many times per day?
12. What chronic diseases have you been diagnosed with?

Right Outlook

13. Rate your overall health.
14. Over the last year, how has your health changed?
15. During the past 30 days, how many days have you felt sad or depressed?
16. During the past 30 days, how many days have you felt worried, tense, or anxious?
17. During the past 30 days, how many days have you felt angry at least once?

Move Naturally

18. On an average day, how many minutes are you physically active?
19. Do you ever take medication to sleep?
20. On average, how many hours do you sleep per night?

Eat Wisely

21. During the past seven days, how many servings of fresh vegetables did you consume?
22. During the past seven days, how many servings of fruit did you consume?
23. During the past seven days, how many servings of unprocessed grains did you consume?
24. During the past seven days, how many servings of beans did you consume?
25. During the past seven days, how many servings of nuts did you consume?
26. During the past seven days, how many servings of fish or seafood did you consume?
27. During the past seven days, how many servings of meat did you consume?
28. During the past seven days, how many servings of dairy products did you consume?
29. During the past seven days, how many servings of sweets did you consume?
30. During the past seven days, how many servings of salty snacks did you consume?

31. During the past seven days, how many meals did you eat at a fast-food chain?

32. During the past seven days, on average, how many alcoholic beverages per day did you consume?

Belong

33. What best describes your relationship status?

34. How satisfied are you with your relationship with your spouse or partner?

35. How satisfied are you with your work life?

36. During the past seven days, how many times did you socialize with people you like?

37. In the past seven days, how many days have you attended religious activities?

Environment

38. How many minutes does it take to get from your home to the closest store that sells fresh produce?

RECORD YOUR RESULTS HERE:

Week 1: _____

Week 4: _____

True Happiness Test

The Blue Zones True Happiness Test, based on the leading scientific research into well-being, will give you a baseline read on where you are at the start of the four weeks. The test was created in cooperation with experts at the University of Pennsylvania World Well-Being Project. By entering your email, you will receive personalized recommendations for how to improve your environment to maximize your happiness. Do this at the beginning and the end of the four weeks. Tracking helps you stay focused.

To receive your personalized recommendations, you will need to take the test online at apps.bluezones.com/en/happiness. The entire test takes five minutes.

HAPPINESS

Here are the questions you will be asked:

Background

1. What year were you born?
2. Sex: male or female?
3. Where do you live?
4. What is your ethnicity?
5. What is your annual household income from all sources?
6. What was the last year of school you completed?

Emotions & Self-Image

7. Rate: I feel positive most of the time.
8. Rate: I feel happy most of the time.
9. Rate: I feel good most of the time.
10. In general, to what extent do you lead a purposeful and meaningful life?
11. If 10 is your best possible life and 1 is the worst, where would you say you stand now?

Environment & Behavior

12. How many vacation days do you take per year?
13. Do you cohabitate with a partner you love and like?
14. How confident are you that you could survive not having a paycheck for a year?
15. On average, how well rested do you feel each day?
16. For how many hours per week do you meditate or

practice other nonreligious relaxation techniques such as tai chi or yoga?

17. On average, how often do you laugh throughout the day?

18. Do you eat at least six servings of fruits or vegetables daily?

19. Rate your overall health.

20. How many hours per week do you volunteer or do work for your community?

21. Do you feel you are part of something greater than yourself (whether that is as a member of a sports team/club, spiritual group, or something else)?

22. How often do you engage in sexual activities?

23. Do you have children?

24. To what extent do you find meaning and significance in your work?

25. If asked, could you explain your sense of life's purpose in a phrase or sentence?

26. How many friends do you have with whom you can have a meaningful conversation or call on a bad day?

27. During the past seven days, how many times did you socialize with people you like?

28. On an average day, how many minutes are you physically active?

29. Do you own a dog?

30. Do you live/work in a place free of traffic noise?

31. Do you visit a dentist at least once per year?

32. How often do you access nature (e.g., walk in a park, hike in a forest, etc.)?

33. To what extent do you have clear life goals and are making progress towards them?

34. How many hours do you do housework in a day?

35. How many minutes do you commute in a car during workdays?

36. Do you care for a loved one who requires your help (e.g., a disabled child or an aging parent)?

RECORD YOUR RESULTS HERE:

Week 1: _____

Week 4: _____

Purpose

Take the Purpose Checkup and put aside some time to write your Purpose Statement. Follow the guide below to unlock your purpose and write your personalized statement.

What Is Purpose?

In the world's blue zones, purpose has always played a

major role in well-being and the resulting extreme longevity. Okinawans call it *ikigai,* or "reason for being." Costa Ricans call it *plan de vida.* Most commonly, though, it's simply referred to as your life's purpose. It's believed that the strong sense of purpose possessed by elders in blue zones regions may act as a buffer against stress and help reduce overall inflammation, in turn lowering chances of suffering from Alzheimer's disease, arthritis, and stroke. There continues to be a growing body of research to support the impact of purpose on mental and physical health and how it can lead to longer life expectancy.

Dr. Robert Butler, the first director of the National Institute on Aging, estimated that an ability to define your life's meaning adds to your life expectancy. Dr. Butler and collaborators led a National Institutes of Health–funded study that looked at the correlation between having a sense of purpose and longevity. His study found that individuals who expressed a clear goal in life—something to get up for in the morning, something that made a difference—lived longer and were sharper than those who did not.

Richard Leider, founder of Inventure—The Purpose Company, and ranked by *Forbes* as one of the top five most respected executive coaches, developed the Purpose Checkup and Guide to Unlocking Your Purpose. This two-step process unlocks your purpose to reveal your lifelong gifts, passions, and values, then helps you create a clear Purpose Statement that energizes you to get up each morning with intention and joy.

Purpose Checkup

Read each statement below carefully and take a few moments to decide on a true response for yourself. Then write the number that most nearly reflects that response. The answers offer the following range of responses:

0: Can't Decide
1: Definitely Disagree
2: Somewhat Disagree
3: Somewhat Agree
4: Definitely Agree

Having (Outer Life): The dimension of your external experience and activity—how effectively you relate to "having" choices in your life.

____ I wake up energized about the day ahead.
____ I feel good about my life and grateful for what I have.
____ I have taken risks to do things I care about.
____ I have found ways to offer my gifts and talents to the world.
____ I'm excited and hopeful about the future.
____ I don't have many regrets about things I haven't done.
____ I go to sleep at night feeling that my day was well lived.

Total Having Score: _____

Doing (Inner Life): The dimension of your internal experience and inner activity—how effectively you relate to the "doing" in your life.

__ Doing things for others is important to me and I make time for it.

__ When I have key decisions to make, I focus on what deeply matters to me and let that be my guide.

__ I enjoy being alone.

__ I know what I'm good at and I use my gifts to make a difference in people's lives.

__ I have the courage to face my adversities.

__ I'm growing and giving.

__ I maintain a balance of saving and savoring the world.

Total Doing Score: _____

Being (Spiritual Life): The dimension of your invisible experience and spiritual activity—how effectively you relate to the "being" choices in your life.

__ I sense the presence of a Higher Power.

__ I maintain a consistent spiritual practice.

__ I feel a sense of the sacred when I'm in the natural world.

__ I offer compassion to others readily.

__ I offer forgiveness to others easily.

__ I feel a deep sense of gratitude for my life.

__ I know what I'd like to be remembered for.

Total Being Score: _____

Total Purpose Checkup Score: _____

Scoring

Your score in each section is one measurement of your development in that dimension. Your total purpose checkup score (out of 84) gives a measure of the power of purpose you are experiencing in your life at present.

- 64–84: Yes, living purposefully! You're clear about what truly matters to you and you're mattering in the world.
- 43–63: Yes, basically fulfilled! Keep on growing and giving in your life.
- 22–42: Unlocking purpose requires more clarity. The next step: Clarify your gifts, passions, and values.
- 0–21: Living purposefully isn't reserved for the elite few. So don't give up because your score right now is low. The power-of-purpose process works, if you work the process!

Guide to Unlocking Your Purpose

There are no rigid formulas for how to write your Purpose Statement, but there are many helpful techniques to assist you. Here are seven mind-changing ideas, developed by Dr. Richard Leider, that have brought powerful results to many people over the years. Use them to see what you can discover about yourself and your dreams.

1. Think about this sentence for a moment: "From family and friends who knew me when I was very young, I have heard that my 'special gifts' are _____." How have these "gifts" persisted in your life?

   _____

   _____

   _____

   _____

   _____

   _____

   _____

2. Imagine being on your deathbed, still clear and coherent, when your best friend drops in to visit you. Your friend asks, "Did you give and receive love?" "Were you authentically you?" "Did you make a small difference in the world?" How would you answer the questions?

_____

_____

_____

_____

_____

_____

_____

_____

_____

3. Get out your calculator and do some "life math." Multiply your age times 365: _____. Then, subtract that number from 30,000, an average life expectancy. Divide that number by 365. Once you get clear that you have _____ more years to wake up, it might inspire you to live more courageously now. How do you feel about how you are spending your most precious currency—your time?

_____

_____

_____

_____

_____

_____

_____

_____

_____

4. How did you wake up this morning? Did you resist getting up, or did you get out of bed with energy and purpose? Think about the way you wake up these days and you will learn something about your life's purpose. What is your "mood" getting up most days?

_____

_____

_____

_____

_____

_____

_____

_____

5. Write the question "What are my gifts?" on five index cards. Give a card to five people who know you well and ask them to write their response to the question on the card. Put the cards all together in a place where you can see them. What theme or thread do you find?

_____

_____

_____

_____

_____

_____

_____

6. Are you curious? What are you most curious about these days? Here are some clues that will help you answer:

   a. Time passes quickly when you're exploring this.
   b. It's so interesting, you can't help spending time on it!
   c. A bad day doing this is better than a good day doing most other things.

7. Look around you for potential models and mentors. Ask yourself who is really leading the kind of life and doing the kind of work that you envision in the next phase of your life. Initiate a courageous conversation to find out: What do they like "most" and "least" about their work?

   _____

   _____

   _____

   _____

   _____

   _____

   _____

   _____

   _____

   _____

These are just some prompts to get you started unlocking your purpose and writing your Purpose Statement. Visit Richard Leider's full guide with more strategies at richardleider.com/wp-content/uploads/2018/08/Power _Of_Purpose.pdf.

POWER OF PURPOSE

Your Purpose Statement

The words in your Purpose Statement must be yours. They must capture your essence. And they must call you to action each and every day. You must envision the impact you'll have on your world as a result of living your purpose. Your actions—not your words—are, ultimately, what truly matters.

I get up in the morning to:

_____

_____

_____

_____

_____

_____

_____

_____

_____

_____

_____

_____

_____

_____

_____

_____

I gain a sense of purpose when:

_____

_____

_____

_____

_____

_____

_____

_____

_____

_____

_____

_____

_____

_____

_____

_____

_____

_____

_____

_____

_____

_____

_____

_____

_____

Find a Blue Zones Buddy or Create a *Moai*

This is not a book about changing habits; it's a book about changing your surroundings to help you live longer and better mindlessly.

Over the next month, the more dimensions of your surroundings you can optimize, the easier it is going to be for you to make unconsciously better decisions as you move through the day. Most of the things we're going to ask you to do this month are going to be easy. Some, however, are going to be difficult. For instance, placing a Post-it Note on your refrigerator reminding you of the foods to never bring into your house is easy. But making a few new friends who will have a huge impact on your health and happiness might be more challenging.

Healthy behaviors (and unhealthy ones) are as contagious as the cold and flu. The people you surround yourself with influence your behaviors, so choose friends who have healthy habits.

The social networks of long-lived people have favorably shaped their health behaviors. A 2018 study at North Carolina State University of more than 700 people found that participants in a weight loss study who enrolled with a buddy lost more weight than those who did it alone.

> A study by the American Society for Training and Development found that if you have a specific accountability appointment with another person you've committed to, you increase your chance of success in completing a goal by 95 percent.

Find at Least One Blue Zones Buddy

Get at least one person to join you in this journey. It would be a fun and easy project to do with people you live with, if a family member or your roommate is on board. People you see regularly such as co-workers, people in your congregation, or neighbors would also make good potential group members. If you can't find anyone you know to join you, ask your friends and family to think about people *they* might know who might be in for the challenge with you. For the best results, find at least one buddy who you can meet with a couple of times a week *in person*. However, if this proves challenging, then reach out to your larger network of friends who may live farther away. A Blue Zones buddy that you "meet" with virtually or via email or Facetime is much better than no buddy at all.

1. Search for the *right* Blue Zones buddy.

Finding the right person to be your buddy is important. It might be better if it's not your best friend or your partner—especially if they won't dive headfirst into this challenge with you. Take a moment to consider people you know. The healthier, the better. You want a partner who will keep you committed and will bring out your best.

If you don't have any healthy friends and you don't have any good referrals for friends of friends, here are some places you might find them:

- Your church, temple, or other faith community. Is there a message board where you can post a notice?
- Plant-based cooking classes
- A volunteer organization that appeals to you. You can connect around shared interests.
- The Blue Zones Life Facebook page
- Try Meetup, a popular and easy-to-use free community group website, or connect with neighbors through a local Facebook group or a site like Nextdoor.
- Neighbors can be the best candidates for Blue Zones buddies. Why? They live close to you and are more likely to be a regular companion. Host a Blue Zones dinner party or Wine @ 5 event and invite your health-minded neighbors. Tell them you're taking the Blue Zones Challenge and invite them to join.

2. Make the connection.

Once you've identified someone who you think might be an ideal buddy, reach out directly. Here's a sample note you can send via email:

Over the next month, I'm taking the Blue Zones Challenge to shape my surroundings to live a longer, better life. Blue zones are places where people live the longest, and one of the secrets to living to 100 is surrounding yourself with healthy, happy people and doing things with them. Research shows that health and happiness are measurably contagious. Since you are [one of the healthiest, happiest people I know/also looking to be healthier and happier], I'm wondering if you'd join me on this monthlong journey. I think we'll both learn something and have some fun along the way. What does this mean? I'm hoping we can walk together a few times a week or get together for healthy meals.

3. Pick a day, time, and way to meet regularly.

While it would be optimal to meet at least once or twice in person each week, a 10-minute daily video chat or phone check-in will also work if you don't live close to your buddy.

Or Create a *Moai*

If you're part of a book club, sports team, or other group, see if you can get everyone to do the Blue Zones Challenge together.

Moai—which roughly means "meeting for a common purpose"—comes from Okinawa, Japan, where the practice originated as a means of social, emotional, and financial support (see page 45).

How to Start a *Moai:*

- Invite four to eight people to join your *moai.*
- Select an activity: walking (or moving naturally) *moai* or potluck *moai.*
- Pick a start date you all agree on and then choose a day and time to meet at least once a week (twice or more is better).
- Create a way for you all to stay in touch regularly, even outside your meet-ups. This can be through a group email, text chain, closed Facebook group, or within an app like WhatsApp so that your members can easily and regularly communicate.
- If doing a walking *moai*, choose routes, trails, or neighborhoods to walk.
- If doing a potluck *moai*, decide who will host the first event and other future locations (parks, etc.). For your potlucks, we recommend you get together and share Blue Zones recipes, but many potluck groups also go out to dinner once in a while to enjoy Wine @ 5 or other Blue Zones–friendly meals.

Extend Your Support Group

Tell people! Even if those around you are not participating, you are more likely to succeed if you make a public announcement of your goals. Be open about starting the Blue Zones Challenge with your family, friends, and co-workers. If your colleagues know that you are cutting out foods like sweets and soda, they might bring you some nuts instead of a candy bar when they make a pit stop at the vending machine. The same goes for your family and friends when they are planning dinner parties or choosing a restaurant venue.

Extend your support team to social media and faraway friends. Share photos of your experiences or tracking sheets on social media. Or send a text at the end of the day to your buddies.

Stay Connected

Join our private Blue Zones Life Facebook group to connect with fellow participants, keep motivated, and remind yourself that everyone is in this for a better life, no matter the speed bumps.

Share photos of your wins, your meals, and your experiences on social media using #mybluezoneslife.

How to Make Friends as an Adult

Just like with dating, making friends as an adult means putting yourself out there. A recent study found that most adults hadn't added to their social circle in five years. So you actually have to get out of the house, and then also ask people out (as friends).

Think about the things you like about yourself and the things that you want to do more of. You want to make friends, but you also want to make friends who will genuinely support you and join you on your journey to a happy, healthy, purpose-filled Blue Zones life. Taking this inventory will help you as you meet new people.

Be likable. Listen and don't hog the conversation. Don't talk over people. Ask questions. Compliment genuinely and often. Put your phone down when you're in a social setting and move away if you need to use it. Give people your undivided attention.

Volunteer in your community for a cause that you care about and that speaks to you. If it's something you do weekly or monthly, hopefully you will see and meet people with like-minded interests.

Look around your existing network and see if there is potential to deepen casual connections. If you're a parent, is there another parent whom you see at school drop-off that seems to have good energy? Or a co-worker whom you banter with? Chat them up. Then see below for how to ask them out on a friend date.

Ask for setups. If you've recently moved, then ask anyone you know if they might have friends in your new area that you might hit it off with. Then ask them to connect you.

Join a social group like a book club, a sports league, a Meetup group around one of your hobbies, or a faith-based group. Danes are among the happiest people in the world, and 92 percent of them are members of a social group.

Take a class. If you've always wanted to try something, take a class that meets regularly.

Try an app. Bumble BFF and Hey! VINA (for women) are just two apps that are like "Tinder for friends."

How to Ask a Friend Out

Make the first move. Say something casual but direct. Try: "Would you want to get coffee or lunch sometime?" If you feel really awkward, then acknowledge it with, "This is awkward, but I'm asking you on a friend date!" If it's someone you don't know well, then ask them for their phone number to finalize plans and keep in touch.

Make it low commitment. Keep it simple and safe and easy. If it's a co-worker, you can ask them to grab lunch. For other people, a coffee or tea or drink is good to start.

If it seems like there's friend chemistry, then don't take too long to schedule the next friend date. It takes a while to get into a rhythm.

Make a group date. If you really find it too awkward to ask someone out on a friend date, then invite them to a casual gathering or outing with one or two other people. Hopefully they will feel flattered to have been asked, and it takes the pressure off the "getting to know you" aspect of a one-on-one meeting.

Know when to move on. If you ask someone to hang out three times and it's a no-go, move on and don't take it personally. If you realize you don't have a lot in common or you don't really have chemistry, then there's nothing wrong with letting people go back into the acquaintance zone.

Walking

"If you want to go fast, walk alone; if you want to go far, walk together." —African proverb

Walking is one of the safest, easiest, and cheapest ways to move naturally throughout the day. Just walking 30 minutes a day can have a big impact on your health and mood.

Even though you can walk alone (and we do suggest you walk as much as you can every day!), one of the foundations of blue zones communities around the world is strong social connections.

Walking with a buddy or a group integrates both the movement and the social aspect of the Blue Zones life.

Research published in the *American Journal of Preventive Medicine* shows people are more likely to walk for recreation or exercise when they are in the company of others or with their pet. Walking and talking is a way to connect while reaping the benefits of moving.

Whether you get a walking buddy or join a walking group, the goal is to meet and walk at least once per week (but more often is better).

Walking is a cost-effective and accessible exercise that can help prevent heart disease, depression, and obesity. Besides the healthful aspects of walking, it also helps you to:

- See your neighborhood, town, and city in a new way.
- Explore local parks and trails safely.
- Make new friend and community connections.

Set Up Your Home

Trying to change your behavior without changing your environment will lead to failure. Now is the time to set up your home and your kitchen for success.

In the Kitchen

You will have a much easier time following the Four Always, Four to Avoid foods and the Blue Zones Food Guidelines if you don't have candy on your counter and a pantry filled with chips and soda. We're not telling you to never have this kind of food, but please don't bring it into your house.

Prepare to make this transition easy by posting the visual guides and decluttering your pantry, kitchen, and refrigerator: Physically remove foods that are off-limits or might be too tempting, such as candies or junk and processed items, and clear your countertops of any kinds of snack foods (that open bag of chips, the box of crackers).

Most of us are on a "see-food diet": We tend to eat what we see. Create an inconvenient junk food cabinet or drawer that is up high or down low. Research shows that if it's out of sight and inconvenient, we'll eat less of it! Finally, put your toaster away and out of sight. A toaster on the counter provides a visual cue to toast something every time you walk into the kitchen, and most of what we put in toasters is unhealthy.

- Remove the Avoid foods from your house: Throw out the soda and other sugar-sweetened beverages, candy, chips, cookies, bacon, and sausages. (You might have to hide these or put them on a top shelf if your family members protest.)
- Stock up on the Always foods like beans, nuts, grains, fruits, and vegetables. We always prefer dried beans and fresh vegetables, but low-sodium, canned versions are okay too. (See page 146 for how to cook dried beans.) Although less processed whole grains like brown rice, barley, and quinoa are better,

100 percent whole-grain products like whole wheat bread and whole wheat pastas are okay too.

- Put a bowl of fresh fruit on your counter.
- Do some meal planning for the week so that grocery shopping is easy.

You can also go full throttle and subscribe to the Blue Zones Meal Planner at meals.bluezones.com (get $20 off a yearly subscription with the code LONGEVITY20).

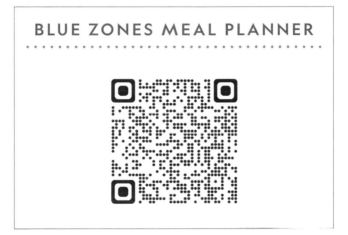

BLUE ZONES MEAL PLANNER

Hang Up the Four Always, Four to Avoid in Your Kitchen

Based on our research with blue zones centenarians, we created these simple food guidelines to help people live better. Although the blue zones longevity hot spots were in very different parts of the world, their residents had similar eating patterns and lifestyles. The longest-lived people in the world ate a plant-slant diet full of beans, whole grains, fruits, veggies, and seeds for almost their whole lives. Nuts were a daily snack, and no processed foods were eaten. Meat was a condiment or a celebratory food in four of the five blue zones; centenarians in one of the blue zones regions were mostly vegetarian.

These are the four best foods to always have on hand and the four worst foods to avoid. The Always foods are readily available, affordable, taste good, and are versatile enough to include in most meals. The Avoid foods are those highly correlated with obesity, heart disease, or cancer, as well as constant temptations in the standard American diet.

Always: 100 Percent Whole Grains (choose farro, quinoa, barley, brown rice, oatmeal, whole cornmeal, bulgur wheat, etc.)

About 65 percent of the diets in the blue zones of the world is whole grains, beans, and starchy tubers. Whole grains include oats, barley, brown rice, and grown corn. Meta-analysis reviews (studies of studies) found that consuming whole grains reduces your risk of diseases that shorten your life. One published in the *British Medical Journal* analyzed 45 studies and concluded that whole grains can help you live longer by cutting your risk of heart disease, cancer, diabetes, respiratory disease, and infectious diseases.

Always: Nuts (variety is good; avoid sugary coatings)

Eat two handfuls of nuts per day. A handful of nuts weighs about two ounces, the average amount that blue zones centenarians consume—almonds in Ikaria and Sardinia, pistachios in Nicoya, and all nuts with the Adventists. The Adventist Health Study found that nut eaters outlive non–nut eaters by an average of two to three years.

Always: Beans (a cup of cooked beans per day)

Beans and legumes are the cornerstone of every longevity diet in the world: black beans in Nicoya; lentils, garbanzo, and white beans in the Mediterranean; and soybeans in Okinawa. People in the blue zones eat at least four times as many beans as Americans do on average.

Always: Fruit & Vegetables (five to 10 servings per day)

According to research published in the *American Journal of Clinical Nutrition*, people who ate five fruits and vegetables a day lived an extra three years compared to their non-plant-eating counterparts. Eating seven or more portions of fruit and veggies a day can lower your risk of premature death by a whopping 42 percent, according to a study published in the *Journal of Epidemiology & Community Health*. But seven is not the upper limit—the protective benefits increase with higher fruit and vegetable consumption.

Plant foods don't just add years to your life, they also directly affect your chronic disease risk. According to a study published in *Nutrition*, even eating two and a half standard portions of fruit and vegetables per day is associated with a 16 percent reduced risk of heart disease, an 18 percent reduced risk of stroke, a 13 percent reduced risk of cardiovascular disease, a 4 percent reduced risk of cancer, and a 15 percent reduction in the risk of premature death.

Avoid: Sugar-Sweetened Beverages

These are unneeded empty calories and the number one source of refined sugars in the American diet.

Avoid: Salty Snacks

Not only are salty snacks high in sodium, they're also fattening. Salty snacks are one of the foods most associated with obesity.

Avoid: Packaged Sweets

Cookies, candies, and processed sweets are also highly associated with obesity.

Avoid: Processed Meats

The World Health Organization puts processed meats in the same category as cigarette smoking—a known carcinogen.

Find a printable version for the Four Always, Four to Avoid at bluezones.com/wp-content/uploads/2019/01/Four-to -Always-Four-to-Avoid.pdf or use the QR code below.

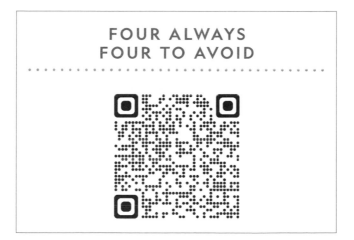

FOUR ALWAYS
FOUR TO AVOID

Four Always, Four to Avoid

✓ FOUR ALWAYS

- -

100% whole grains:
Brown rice, farro, quinoa, bulgar, oatmeal, cornmeal.

Nuts:
A handful a day.

Beans:
A cup of beans per day.

Fruit & vegetables:
5-10 servings per day.

✗ FOUR TO AVOID

- -

Sugar-sweetened beverages:
Empty calories.

Salty snacks:
Too much salt and preservatives.

Packaged sweets:
Cookies, candies, donuts, and processed sweets.

Processed meats:
Linked to cancer and heart disease.

Post the Blue Zones Food Guidelines in Your Kitchen

We distilled more than 150 dietary surveys of the world's longest-lived people to discover the secrets of a longevity diet.

These 11 simple guidelines reflect how the world's longest-lived people ate for most of their lives. We make it easy to eat like the healthiest people in the world with the Blue Zones Meal Planner, where you'll find thousands of recipes that follow these guidelines, making plant-slant food delicious and accessible. By adopting some of the healthy eating principles into your daily life, you too can Live Longer, Better®. Head to bluezones.com/recipes/food-guidelines or use the QR code below to download our free printable of the Blue Zones Food Guidelines so you can post it in your home as a daily reminder.

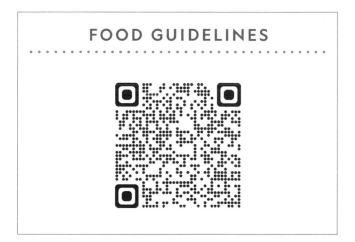

FOOD GUIDELINES

Aim for a 95 to 100 percent plant-based diet.

People in the blue zones eat an impressive variety of garden vegetables when they are in season, and then they pickle or dry the surplus to enjoy during the off-season. The best-of-the-best longevity foods are leafy greens such as spinach, kale, beet and turnip tops, chard, and collards. Combined with seasonal fruits and vegetables, whole grains, and beans, they dominate blue zones meals all year long.

Many oils derive from plants, and they are all preferable to animal-based fats. We cannot say that olive oil is the only healthy plant-based oil, but it is the one most often used in the blue zones. Evidence shows that olive oil consumption increases good cholesterol and lowers bad cholesterol. In Ikaria, we found that for middle-age people, about six tablespoons of olive oil daily seemed to cut the risk of dying in half.

People in four of the five blue zones consume meat, but they do so sparingly, using it as a celebratory food, a small side, or a way to flavor dishes. Research suggests that 30-year-old vegetarian Adventists will likely outlive their meat-eating counterparts by as many as eight years. At the same time, increasing the amount of plant-based foods in your meals has many salutary effects. Beans, greens, yams and sweet potatoes, fruits, nuts, and seeds should all be favored. Whole grains are okay too. Try a variety of fruits and vegetables; know which ones you like, and keep your kitchen stocked with them.

Retreat from meat.

Averaging out consumption in blue zones, we found that people ate about two ounces of meat or less about five times per month. And we don't know if they lived longer despite eating meat.

The Adventist Health Study 2, which has been following 96,000 Americans since 2002, has found that the people who live the longest are vegans or pesco-vegetarians who eat a plant-based diet that includes a small amount of fish.

So we don't recommend meat consumption. Okinawans probably offer the best meat substitute: extra firm tofu, high in protein and cancer-fighting phytoestrogens.

Go easy on fish.

If you must eat fish, eat fewer than three ounces, up to three times weekly. In most blue zones, people ate some fish but less than you might think—up to three small servings a week. There are other ethical and health considerations involved in including fish in your diet. It makes sense, for example, to select fish that are common and abundant, not threatened by overfishing. In the world's blue zones, in most cases, the fish being eaten are small, relatively inexpensive fish such as sardines, anchovies, and cod—middle-of-the-food-chain species that are not exposed to the high levels of mercury or other chemicals like PCBs that pollute our gourmet fish supply today.

Fish is not a necessary part of a longevity diet, but if you must eat seafood, select fish that are common and not threatened by overfishing.

Reduce dairy.

Milk from cows doesn't figure significantly in any blue zones diet except that of some Adventists. Arguments against milk often focus on its high fat and sugar content. The number of people who (often unknowingly) have some difficulty digesting lactose may be as high as 60 percent. Goat's and sheep's milk products figure into the Ikarian and Sardinian blue zones.

Eliminate eggs.

Though people in the blue zones eat some eggs, we don't recommend them. Consumption of eggs has been correlated to higher rates of prostate cancer for men and exacerbated kidney problems for women. Some people with heart or circulatory problems choose to forgo eggs. Again, eggs aren't necessary for living a long life. Moreover, people with diabetes should be cautious of eating egg yolks.

Get a daily dose of beans.

Eat at least a half cup of cooked beans daily. Beans, legumes, and pulses reign supreme in blue zones.

The fact is, beans are the consummate superfood. On average, they are made up of 21 percent protein, 77 percent complex carbohydrates (the kind that deliver a slow and steady energy rather than the spike you get from refined carbohydrates like white flour), and only a few percent fat. They are also an excellent source of fiber. They're cheap and versatile, come in a variety of textures, and are packed with more nutrients per gram than any other food on earth. Beans are a meal staple in all five of the blue zones—with a dietary average of at least a half cup per day, which provides most of the vitamins and minerals you need. And because beans are so hearty and satisfying, they'll likely push less healthy foods out of your diet.

Slash sugar.

Consume only 28 grams (7 teaspoons) of added sugar daily. People in the blue zones eat sugar intentionally, not by habit or accident. They consume about the same amount of naturally occurring sugars as North Americans do, but only a fraction of added sugar—no more than seven teaspoons a day. It's hard to avoid sugar. It occurs naturally in fruits, vegetables, and even milk. But that's not the problem.

Between 1970 and 2000, the amount of added sugar in the American food supply rose by 25 percent. This adds up to about 22 teaspoons of added sugar each of us consumes daily—insidious, hidden sugars mixed into soda, yogurt, and sauces. Too much sugar in our diet has been shown to suppress the immune system. It also spikes insulin levels, which can lead to diabetes and lower fertility, make you fat, and even shorten your life.

Our advice: If you must eat sweets, save cookies, candy, and bakery items for special occasions, ideally as part of a meal. Limit sugar added to coffee, tea, and other foods to no more than four teaspoons per day. Skip any product that lists sugar among its first five ingredients.

Snack on nuts.

Eat two handfuls of nuts per day.

The optimal mix of nuts: almonds (high in vitamin E and magnesium), peanuts (high in protein and folate, a B vitamin), Brazil nuts (high in selenium, a mineral found effective in protecting against prostate cancer), cashews (high in magnesium), and walnuts (high in alpha-linolenic acid, the only omega-3 fat found in a plant-based food). Walnuts, peanuts, and almonds are the nuts most likely to lower your cholesterol.

Sour on bread.

Eat only sourdough or 100 percent whole wheat bread. Blue zones bread is unlike the bread most Americans buy. Most commercially available breads start with bleached white flour, which metabolizes quickly into sugar and spikes insulin levels. But bread from the blue zones is either whole grain or sourdough, each with its own healthful characteristics. In Ikaria and Sardinia, breads are made from a variety of whole grains such as wheat, rye, and barley, each of which offers a wide spectrum of nutrients, such as tryptophan, an amino acid, and the minerals selenium and magnesium.

Whole grains also have higher levels of fiber than most commonly used wheat flours. Some traditional blue zones breads are made with naturally occurring bacteria called lactobacilli, which "digest" the starches and glutens while making the bread rise. The process also creates an acid— the "sour" in sourdough. The result is bread with less gluten even than breads labeled "gluten free," and with a longer shelf life and a pleasantly sour taste that most people like. Traditional sourdough breads actually lower the glycemic load of meals, making your entire meal healthier, slower burning, easier on your pancreas, and more likely to make calories available as energy than stored as fat.

Go wholly whole.

Choose foods that are recognizable. People in blue zones traditionally eat the whole food. They don't throw the yolk away to make an egg-white omelet, or spin the fat out of their yogurt, or juice the fiber-rich pulp out of their fruits. They also don't enrich or add extra ingredients to change the nutritional profile of their foods. Instead of taking vitamins or other supplements, they get everything they need from nutrient-dense, fiber-rich whole foods.

A good definition of a "whole food" would be one that is made of a single ingredient, raw, cooked, ground, or fermented, and not highly processed. Tofu is minimally processed, for example, while cheese-flavored corn puffs are highly processed. Blue zones dishes typically contain a half dozen or so ingredients, simply blended together.

Almost all of the foods consumed by centenarians in the blue zones grow within a 10-mile radius of their homes. They eat raw fruits and vegetables; they grind whole grains themselves, and then cook them slowly. They use fermentation—an ancient way to make nutrients bio-available—in the tofu, sourdough bread, wine, and pickled vegetables they eat. And they rarely ingest artificial preservatives.

Drink mostly water.

Never drink soft drinks (including diet soda). With very few exceptions, people in blue zones drink coffee, tea, water, and wine. Period. (Soft drinks, which account for about half of Americans' sugar intake, were unknown to most blue zones centenarians.) There is a strong rationale for each.

- Water: Adventists recommend seven glasses of water daily. They point to studies that show that being hydrated facilitates blood flow and lessens the chance of a blood clot.

- Coffee: Sardinians, Ikarians, and Nicoyans all drink copious amounts of coffee. Research associates coffee drinking with lower rates of dementia and Parkinson's disease.

- Tea: People in all the blue zones drink tea. Okinawans nurse green tea all day. Green tea has been shown to lower the risk of heart disease and several cancers. Ikarians drink brews of rosemary, wild sage, and dandelion—all herbs known to have anti-inflammatory properties.

- Red wine: People who drink—in moderation— tend to outlive those who don't. (This doesn't mean you should start drinking if you don't drink now.) People in most blue zones drink one to three small glasses of red wine per day, often with a meal and with friends.

Make Movement Natural

In Sight, in Mind

Make it easy to bike or walk more. Buy comfortable shoes or put your running or walking shoes out where you can see them. Try by the front door, even though they probably won't go with your décor. You're more likely to take that walk if your shoes are set out where you can see and easily access them, rather than having to hunt them down in the back of a closet.

If you're investing in a new pair of sneakers, get the best quality you can afford and try to visit a running store to get advice on the best shoes for your feet and your running or walking style.

If you buy a bike or fix your current bike, then do the same for other family members so you can ride together. Use good-quality helmets to prevent injury.

Food Guidelines

BLUE ZONES™

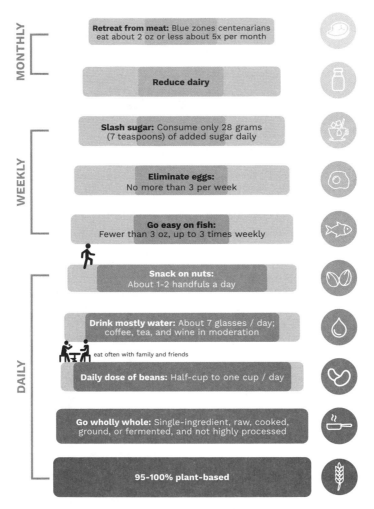

MONTHLY

Retreat from meat: Blue zones centenarians eat about 2 oz or less about 5x per month

Reduce dairy

WEEKLY

Slash sugar: Consume only 28 grams (7 teaspoons) of added sugar daily

Eliminate eggs: No more than 3 per week

Go easy on fish: Fewer than 3 oz, up to 3 times weekly

DAILY

Snack on nuts: About 1-2 handfuls a day

Drink mostly water: About 7 glasses / day; coffee, tea, and wine in moderation

eat often with family and friends

Daily dose of beans: Half-cup to one cup / day

Go wholly whole: Single-ingredient, raw, cooked, ground, or fermented, and not highly processed

95-100% plant-based

CENTENARIANS
IN THE BLUE ZONES

Although the centenarians in the blue zones did eat some meat, we are asking you to go 100 percent plant-based during this month. We know in your "normal" life, you probably eat animal products. Research does show that the closer you can get to a whole-food, plant-based diet, the less likely you are to develop heart disease, dementia, diabetes, and several types of cancer. This month, we really want you to cleanse your diet of meat, dairy, and processed foods. We believe that you'll lose weight, lower your cholesterol and blood pressure, and maybe even reverse your prediabetes. Also, since high-fat foods like animal products and snack foods napalm your taste buds, you'll find that you'll enjoy the subtle flavors and textures that plant-based foods provide even more without meat. To learn more about what happens in a day, week, and month when you eat a plant-based diet, go to bluezones.com /plantbased.

Why do it: People who live in blue zones areas use active transportation. You easily incorporate physical activity into your daily life if you own running shoes or a bike and put them in a spot where you'll be reminded to use them.

On the Floor, Not the Couch

Okinawa, Japan, is one of the five blue zones where elders live exceptionally long and healthy lives. Traditionally, Okinawan people sit on the floor to read, eat, talk, and relax instead of sitting in chairs, though this practice is dying out there and among younger generations throughout Asia. Okinawan seniors sit and get up from the floor dozens or hundreds of times per day. This exercises their legs, back, and core in a natural way. Sitting on the floor also improves posture and increases overall strength, flexibility, and mobility. Studies correlate the "ability to sit and rise from the floor without support" with a longer life expectancy. Sitting on the floor also develops musculoskeletal fitness.

Do it yourself! Set up some cushions on the floor and sit there instead of on the couch when you're reading, doing work, talking on the phone, or relaxing. If it's hard for you to go all the way down at first, you can transition by sitting on a medicine ball or a floor chair with a back until your muscles strengthen up.

Why do it: Sitting on the floor works your thighs, glutes, and lower back each time you sit down and stand back up. Supporting yourself without a chairback improves posture and may help you burn up to an additional 130 calories each hour. Okinawans sit on the floor and get up and down all day, every day (even nonagenarians and centenarians!).

Put Your Scale in a Visible Place and Use It Daily

If you don't have a scale, buy an inexpensive one. It doesn't need all the bells and whistles. If you do have one, put it in a convenient place so you'll use it every day.

It's true that your weight is only one indicator of health, and not even the most important. As you build muscle and lose fat, your weight may stay the same, or even increase. But with the Blue Zones Challenge, we still recommend you weigh yourself every day.

Why?

First of all, knowing your weight is a vital factor in successfully losing weight. Research has shown that weighing yourself more often, versus weighing yourself less often, is associated with greater weight loss. Keeping track of your progress can keep you motivated to make healthy decisions related to your weight and overall health.

Checking your weight frequently is correlated to preventing weight gain in the first place. In a study published in the *International Journal of Behavioral Medicine*, if an overweight adult weighed themselves daily throughout a two-year period, they lost 10 pounds. In the same study, if they only weighed themselves monthly, they gained 2.2 pounds.

Bottom line: Put a scale in your way and weigh every day.

In addition to checking the scale, you can track your progress by:

- Tracking fat and muscle mass with a BMI scale.
- Noticing how your clothing is fitting.
- Measuring your waist, and tracking your progress by inches lost.
- Taking pictures of yourself regularly.

Weighing yourself every day might be just the thing you need to stay focused and on track. Remember to take your reading at the same time every day, wearing similar clothing. Morning, after you've gone to the bathroom and before you've had anything to eat or drink, is generally the best time to weigh yourself.

Remember, the point of weighing yourself frequently is to track a trend in your weight. On a daily basis your weight can change due to water retention, PMS and menstruation, and what you ate the day before. So, don't beat yourself up if your weight goes up a little bit. Take a deep breath and watch for things to settle down.

Record Your Progress

	Week 1	Week 2	Week 3	Week 4
Weight				
BMI				
Clothing Size				
Waist				

Tips for Success

Starting a new behavior seems like the hardest part of the process of change, but it's actually maintaining behaviors that is the hardest part. That's why your Blue Zones tasks and activities over the next month will help you create an environment and social circle that are mutually supportive—so that these healthy behaviors aren't work but become the default option.

1. Don't quit.

People can and do put themselves through cabbage diets, soup diets, cleansing diets, and smoothie diets. Those diets are hard to maintain and it's easy to fall off the wagon. The Blue Zones Challenge is not a deprivation diet. We don't expect perfection, but we know that you'll be pleased with your progress if you stick it out—you can do this!

2. Make every day count.

Unlike other programs, the Blue Zones Challenge is about changing your surroundings, not just what's on your plate. This book tries to help you understand the things that helped the world's longest-lived people live so long, and then to set up your life to make it easy for you to replicate their success. Many elements affect our health and longevity, and they often go hand in hand. (If you don't get a good night's rest, it's hard to exercise or eat healthily the next day.) Even if you slip up, try to do as many of the Blue Zones prompts as you can. If you are feeling sick and can't meet up with your walking buddy, make sure to eat your Blue Zones meals and to combine as many of the other Blue Zones Power 9® lessons and activities as you can. Start again tomorrow.

3. Talk about this. Get support. Get help.

People in blue zones live in communities and enjoy village life. If they don't show up to church or the temple or to the village festival, people come knocking on their door. Create your own community circle that will support you through the next few weeks and help you sustain this lifestyle for years to come. And encourage yourself by keeping up with the Blue Zones weekly tracking sheets and materials. Store them in this journal or rip them out and hang them where you can see them and track your progress.

WEEK 1 SCORE

You may not be able to finish all these activities in a week.
If that is the case, feel free to use the rest of the month.

ACTIVITY	POINTS
Found a Blue Zones buddy or created a *moai* who are completing the Challenge with you (30 points)	
Took the Purpose Checkup and wrote Purpose Statement (20 points)	
Took the True Vitality Test and recorded results (15 points)	
Took the True Happiness Test and recorded results (15 points)	
Posted the list of Four Always, Four to Avoid foods in the kitchen (5 points)	
Posted the Blue Zones Food Guidelines in the kitchen (5 points)	
Bought a scale or put mine in a convenient place (5 points)	
Wearing a blue bracelet or other blue jewelry (a ring, watch, etc.) as a reminder of *hara hachi bu* (5 points)	
TOTAL WEEKLY POINTS:	

TARGET FOR THE WEEK = 100 POINTS

Three Big Wins This Week

1. _____
2. _____
3. _____

Lessons I Learned This Week

_____
_____
_____

Gratitude List

_____
_____
_____

Notes/Journaling

_____
_____
_____
_____
_____
_____
_____
_____
_____
_____
_____

GALLO PINTO

Total cook time: 20 minutes | Makes 3 servings

INGREDIENTS

1½ tablespoons vegetable oil

1 onion, chopped

1 clove garlic, minced

2 tablespoons Worcestershire sauce

1½ cups cooked black beans (or one 8-ounce can black beans, drained)

3 cups cooked long-grain white rice

Salt and pepper (optional)

½ avocado, sliced, for topping

Chilero hot sauce (optional as garnish)

Chopped cilantro (optional as garnish)

Sliced mango (optional as garnish)

STEPS

1. In a large skillet, heat the oil over medium heat. Add the onion and sauté until it starts to soften, about 4 minutes.

2. Add the garlic and cook for another 5 to 7 minutes, or until the vegetables are browned.

3. Add the Worcestershire sauce and beans; turn the heat to low and stir. Cook for 2 to 3 minutes more.

4. Add the rice and stir to combine. Cook and stir until the rice and beans are evenly distributed and are heated through. Season with salt and pepper to taste.

5. Top with sliced avocado and, if desired, hot sauce, chopped cilantro, and sliced mango.

BREAKFAST COOKIES

Total cook time: 25 minutes | Makes 4 servings

. . . .

INGREDIENTS

3 large ripe bananas

1¾ cups quick oats

¼ cup chocolate chips

¼ cup applesauce

Honey (optional)

Crushed nuts (optional)

STEPS

1. Preheat the oven to 350 degrees F. Line a baking sheet with parchment paper or grease it with cooking spray.

2. Mash the bananas in a bowl; add the oats and mix well to combine. Fold in the chocolate chips and applesauce.

3. Use a tablespoon to measure out portions of the dough, dropping them onto the baking sheet. You can shape these into balls or press and flatten each cookie with a spoon. (The dough will not spread out much during baking.)

4. Bake for about 15 minutes, or until the cookies are lightly browned on top. Remove and let them cool on a rack.

5. Roll in the honey and then the crushed nuts, if using, when the cookies are cool enough to handle.

SPAGHETTI WITH WALNUT PESTO

Total cook time: 40 minutes | Makes 6 servings

. . . .

INGREDIENTS

¼ cup walnuts

6 quarts water

1 pound spaghetti or linguine

2 large cloves garlic, finely chopped

2 tablespoons chopped fresh Italian parsley

½ cup extra-virgin olive oil

2 tablespoons salt

1 cup (¼ pound) freshly grated pecorino cheese (optional)

STEPS

1. Grind the walnuts in a food processor until chopped but not overprocessed (avoid mincing or forming a paste).

2. In a large pot, bring the 6 quarts of water to a boil. Add the pasta and cook until almost al dente; reserve 1 cup of cooking water, then drain.

3. In a very large sauté pan, cook the nuts, garlic, and parsley in the olive oil over low heat until the garlic is soft, 8 to 9 minutes.

4. Add the pasta and gently mix to combine it with the sauce. Add as much of the reserved cooking water as you need to get the sauce to the consistency you prefer—probably ¼ to ½ cup. Season with salt.

5. If using cheese, add the pecorino to the pasta and serve immediately.

MISO SOUP

Total cook time: 25 minutes | Makes 6 servings

INGREDIENTS

3 tablespoons miso paste, such as shiro miso (white), miso (aka red miso), or shinshu miso (yellow)

1½ tablespoons unseasoned rice wine vinegar

1 large garlic clove, peeled

1¼ inch piece of fresh ginger, peeled

5 cups water, divided

½ pound firm tofu, cut into ½-inch cubes

¼ pound fresh shiitake mushrooms, stemmed and the caps thinly sliced

2 cups pea shoots (about 3 ounces), roughly chopped

6 medium scallions, trimmed and thinly chopped

2 teaspoons toasted sesame oil

1 teaspoon soy sauce

STEPS

1. Put the miso, rice wine vinegar, garlic, ginger, and 1 cup of the water in a food processor or a large blender. Cover and process or blend until smooth, scraping down the inside of the canister at least once.

2. Stir the miso mixture into the 4 remaining cups water in a medium saucepan. Add the tofu, mushrooms, pea shoots, and scallions; bring to a simmer over medium heat, stirring often.

3. Reduce the heat to low and simmer, uncovered, for 5 minutes. Turn off the heat and stir in the sesame oil and soy sauce before serving.

4. Serve with rice.

TIP: If you like more texture, finely mince the garlic and ginger but don't put them in the food processor or blender. Instead, add them with the tofu.

TIP: If fresh shiitake mushrooms are not available, soak 4 large dried shiitakes with warm tap water to cover in a small bowl for 20 minutes. Drain, reserving the soaking liquid. Strain the liquid through cheesecloth to remove any grit. Use this soaking liquid, reducing the amount of water in the saucepan by an equivalent amount.

TIP: Substitute baby spinach or stemmed watercress for the pea shoots.

LEMON AND HERB
ROASTED POTATOES

Total cook time: 1 hour, 15 minutes | Makes 10–12 servings

INGREDIENTS

5 pounds potatoes (Yukon Gold work well), scrubbed and cut into thin wedges

6 cloves garlic, minced

¾ cup olive oil

½ cup good-quality veggie broth

½ cup water

¼ cup freshly squeezed lemon juice

3 teaspoons sea salt, plus more to taste

1 teaspoon freshly ground black pepper, plus more to taste

1 tablespoon dried oregano

1 teaspoon chopped fresh mint

STEPS

1. Preheat the oven to 450 degrees F. Lightly coat a large baking dish in olive oil.

2. In a large bowl, stir the potatoes, garlic, olive oil, broth, water, lemon juice, salt, and pepper together until the potatoes are evenly coated.

3. Pour the potato mixture into the baking dish. Roast in the oven until the potatoes start to brown, about 40 minutes.

4. Remove the potatoes from the oven. Add the oregano and mint to them, stirring to combine. If the potatoes look dry, pour another ½ cup broth into the dish.

5. Return to the oven and bake about 30 minutes longer.

6. Adjust the seasoning with salt and pepper, if needed.

BIG-BATCH ADVENTIST VEGETABLE SOUP

Total cook time: 1 hour | Makes 12 servings

INGREDIENTS

4 carrots, diced

4 to 6 stalks celery, diced

Big handful of diced shallots

½ cup sliced peppers (red or yellow bell peppers work nicely)

2 tablespoons olive oil

4 potatoes, large diced

4 sprigs thyme

4 sprigs oregano

1 teaspoon Better Than Bouillon vegetable base

½ cup carrot juice

12 cups vegetable broth

Large handful of uncooked lentils and/or brown rice

2 to 3 splashes of white or rosé wine, or bourbon (optional)

½ the zest and all the juice of 1 tangerine or small orange

Handful of chopped flat leaf parsley (optional)

STEPS

1. In a large soup pot, sauté the carrots, celery, shallots, and peppers in olive oil over medium-high heat for about 3 minutes.

2. Add all the remaining ingredients except the citrus and parsley to the pot. Raise the heat to bring to a boil, then simmer over medium-low heat for 45 to 50 minutes.

3. Finish by adding the citrus zest and juice, stirring to combine. Add the parsley, if using.

TIP: Customize this soup as you like! You can replace the lentils and/or brown rice with tofu, cooked grains, or pasta toward the end of the cooking time. Peas or edamame are also good additions.

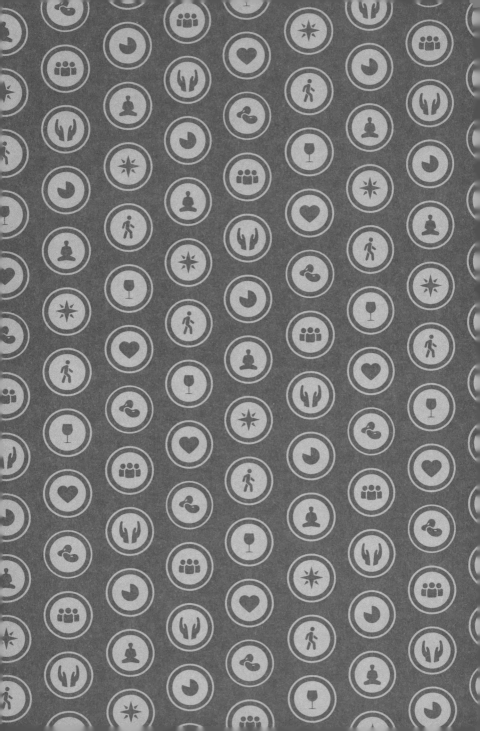

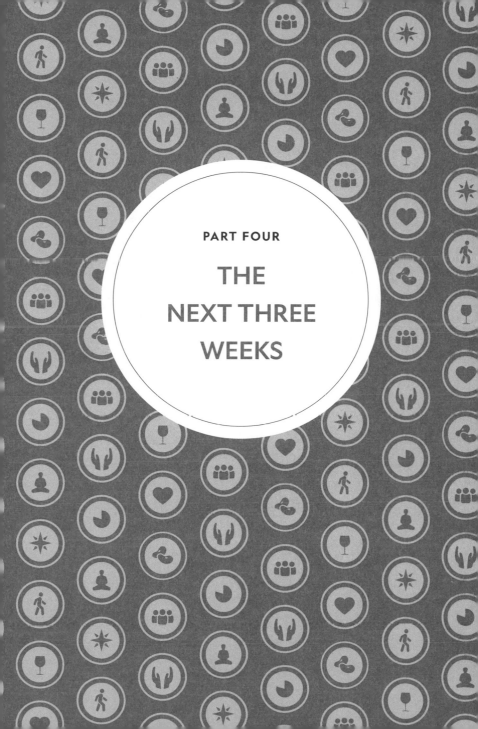

PART FOUR

THE
NEXT THREE
WEEKS

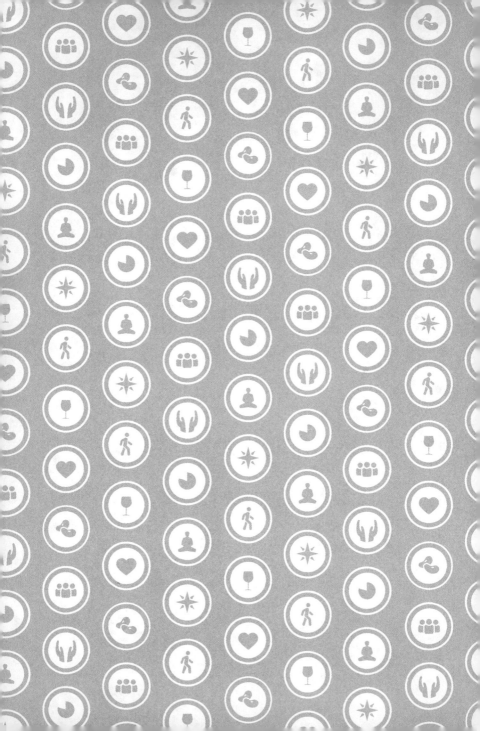

≈

Complete Your 30 Days

N OW THAT YOU'VE SET UP YOUR SURROUNDINGS AND LIFE FOR SUCCESS, you're ready to start the next three weeks of the challenge. You'll be recording your progress every day in this planner.

Recording your tasks or doing any kind of journaling can seem backward and a waste of time. But there's a lot of research that shows it helps with short- and long-term goals. You can review your progress weekly to make sure you are on track, plan for some of your time-intensive tasks as you review your activity, and look back at your progress and celebrate how much you've achieved in such a short amount of time.

The Blue Zones Challenge
WEEK 2

Week 2 Activities

- Put your running shoes or bike out where you can see them (and use them!).
- Start the practice of *hara hachi bu* (stop eating when you are 80 percent full).
- Eat at least three Blue Zones meals this week.
- Walk with your group or buddy at least once.
- If possible, take public transportation to work or to do an errand at least once (p. 143).
- Host a potluck to try out some new Blue Zones recipes.
- Suggest a walking meeting at work (p. 143).
- Fill your fruit bowl with your favorite fruit, and leave it on your counter.
- Limit your workweek to 40 hours.
- Discover an herbal tea you love (p. 141).
- Tape a reminder note to your dashboard (p. 142).
- Install a browser extension or app (p. 142).

WEEKLY BONUS POINTS

ACTIVITY	POINTS
Walked or ate with my *moai* or Blue Zones buddy (3 points each time)	
Volunteered for at least 30 minutes (3 points each time)	
Tried new Blue Zones recipes (goal = 3 recipes) (1 for each recipe)	
Completed other Blue Zones activities this week (2 for each activity)	
Spent at least 30 minutes engaged in a hobby or passion (1 point each time)	

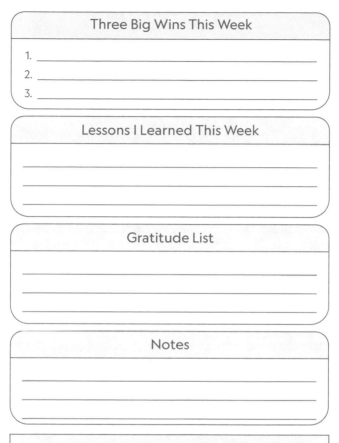

Three Big Wins This Week

1. _____
2. _____
3. _____

Lessons I Learned This Week

_____
_____
_____

Gratitude List

_____
_____
_____

Notes

_____
_____
_____

The Blue Zones Challenge
DAILY CHECK-IN

Track your progress every day to see how you're reshaping your environment, the spaces in which you live, your health, and your happiness. Each of the daily worksheets on the following pages will help you record the activities, foods, and steps you're taking toward a Blue Zones lifestyle. Keep track of how you're doing with the daily scorecard—you should improve each day and week.

DAY 1 SCORECARD

ACTIVITY	POINTS
Ate 100% whole-food, plant-based diet today (5 points)	
Ate a cup of beans today (3 points)	
Consumed all meals / calories within 10-hour window (2 points)	
Walked or did some other physical activity at least 30 minutes today (can be multiple walks) (2 points)	
Screen time less than 1 hour (outside work / school) (2 points)	
Recorded my weight (1 point)	
Recorded what I ate (1 point)	
Servings of poultry, pork, beef, lamb (-1 per serving)	
Servings of cow's milk products (milk, cheese, etc.) (-1 per serving)	
Servings of processed foods (packaged cookies, candies, chips, etc.) (-1 per serving)	
Servings of sweetened beverages (soda, fruit drinks, sport drinks) (-1 per serving)	
DAILY SCORE:	

DAILY TARGET = 12 POINTS A DAY

DAY 2 SCORECARD

ACTIVITY	POINTS
Ate 100% whole-food, plant-based diet today (5 points)	
Ate a cup of beans today (3 points)	
Consumed all meals / calories within 10-hour window (2 points)	
Walked or did some other physical activity at least 30 minutes today (can be multiple walks) (2 points)	
Screen time less than 1 hour (outside work / school) (2 points)	
Recorded my weight (1 point)	
Recorded what I ate (1 point)	
Servings of poultry, pork, beef, lamb (-1 per serving)	
Servings of cow's milk products (milk, cheese, etc.) (-1 per serving)	
Servings of processed foods (packaged cookies, candies, chips, etc.) (-1 per serving)	
Servings of sweetened beverages (soda, fruit drinks, sport drinks) (-1 per serving)	
DAILY SCORE:	

DAILY TARGET = 12 POINTS A DAY

DAY 3 SCORECARD

ACTIVITY	POINTS
Ate 100% whole-food, plant-based diet today (5 points)	
Ate a cup of beans today (3 points)	
Consumed all meals / calories within 10-hour window (2 points)	
Walked or did some other physical activity at least 30 minutes today (can be multiple walks) (2 points)	
Screen time less than 1 hour (outside work / school) (2 points)	
Recorded my weight (1 point)	
Recorded what I ate (1 point)	
Servings of poultry, pork, beef, lamb (-1 per serving)	
Servings of cow's milk products (milk, cheese, etc.) (-1 per serving)	
Servings of processed foods (packaged cookies, candies, chips, etc.) (-1 per serving)	
Servings of sweetened beverages (soda, fruit drinks, sport drinks) (-1 per serving)	
DAILY SCORE:	

DAILY TARGET = 12 POINTS A DAY

DAY 4 SCORECARD

ACTIVITY	POINTS
Ate 100% whole-food, plant-based diet today (5 points)	
Ate a cup of beans today (3 points)	
Consumed all meals / calories within 10-hour window (2 points)	
Walked or did some other physical activity at least 30 minutes today (can be multiple walks) (2 points)	
Screen time less than 1 hour (outside work / school) (2 points)	
Recorded my weight (1 point)	
Recorded what I ate (1 point)	
Servings of poultry, pork, beef, lamb (-1 per serving)	
Servings of cow's milk products (milk, cheese, etc.) (-1 per serving)	
Servings of processed foods (packaged cookies, candies, chips, etc.) (-1 per serving)	
Servings of sweetened beverages (soda, fruit drinks, sport drinks) (-1 per serving)	
DAILY SCORE:	

DAILY TARGET = 12 POINTS A DAY

DAY 5 SCORECARD

ACTIVITY	POINTS
Ate 100% whole-food, plant-based diet today (5 points)	
Ate a cup of beans today (3 points)	
Consumed all meals / calories within 10-hour window (2 points)	
Walked or did some other physical activity at least 30 minutes today (can be multiple walks) (2 points)	
Screen time less than 1 hour (outside work / school) (2 points)	
Recorded my weight (1 point)	
Recorded what I ate (1 point)	
Servings of poultry, pork, beef, lamb (-1 per serving)	
Servings of cow's milk products (milk, cheese, etc.) (-1 per serving)	
Servings of processed foods (packaged cookies, candies, chips, etc.) (-1 per serving)	
Servings of sweetened beverages (soda, fruit drinks, sport drinks) (-1 per serving)	
DAILY SCORE:	

DAILY TARGET = 12 POINTS A DAY

DAY 6 SCORECARD

ACTIVITY	POINTS
Ate 100% whole-food, plant-based diet today (5 points)	
Ate a cup of beans today (3 points)	
Consumed all meals / calories within 10-hour window (2 points)	
Walked or did some other physical activity at least 30 minutes today (can be multiple walks) (2 points)	
Screen time less than 1 hour (outside work / school) (2 points)	
Recorded my weight (1 point)	
Recorded what I ate (1 point)	
Servings of poultry, pork, beef, lamb (-1 per serving)	
Servings of cow's milk products (milk, cheese, etc.) (-1 per serving)	
Servings of processed foods (packaged cookies, candies, chips, etc.) (-1 per serving)	
Servings of sweetened beverages (soda, fruit drinks, sport drinks) (-1 per serving)	
DAILY SCORE:	

DAILY TARGET = 12 POINTS A DAY

DAY 7 SCORECARD

ACTIVITY	POINTS
Ate 100% whole-food, plant-based diet today (5 points)	
Ate a cup of beans today (3 points)	
Consumed all meals / calories within 10-hour window (2 points)	
Walked or did some other physical activity at least 30 minutes today (can be multiple walks) (2 points)	
Screen time less than 1 hour (outside work / school) (2 points)	
Recorded my weight (1 point)	
Recorded what I ate (1 point)	
Servings of poultry, pork, beef, lamb (-1 per serving)	
Servings of cow's milk products (milk, cheese, etc.) (-1 per serving)	
Servings of processed foods (packaged cookies, candies, chips, etc.) (-1 per serving)	
Servings of sweetened beverages (soda, fruit drinks, sport drinks) (-1 per serving)	
DAILY SCORE:	

DAILY TARGET = 12 POINTS A DAY

WEEKLY SCORE BOX

Weekly Score = Daily Totals + Weekly Bonus Points

Week 1: _____ Week 2: _____

Target: 400 points for the whole month

Tips and Tricks

Discover an herbal tea you love.

Black, green, or herbal, we know tea is the longevity drink enjoyed most among the longest-lived people in the world. Older Ikarians show almost no signs of dementia or many of the other chronic illnesses that affect the Western world. Their family values, long-standing traditions, and their love of herbal teas, among other lifestyle factors, allow a third of the Ikarians to live to at least age 90. They drink strong red wine, stay up late, sleep in, and know how to relax. They are active outdoors and in their gardens. They live like mountain people and eat a healthy Mediterranean-style diet. (See page 212 to read about Ikarians' fasting and how you can apply the practice in your own life.)

In addition to their diet rich in beans, wild greens, olive oil, lemons, and potatoes, they frequently brew tea from wild herbs. Greek teas may offer specific beneficial effects: wild mint as a way to prevent gingivitis and ulcers; rosemary to treat gout; artemisia to improve blood circulation.

When I was in Ikaria studying the diets of the longest-lived, healthiest people, I sent samples of Ikarian herbal teas to be laboratory tested and found that they all had antioxidant properties in addition to functioning as mild diuretics. So not only do they contain powerful antioxidants but they can also help flush waste products from the body and slightly lower blood pressure. Discover your favorite, be it rosemary, oregano, mint, sage, or another herb. Then drink it daily.

Tape a reminder note to your dashboard to park as far away as you can from the door.

Our Western lifestyle is sedentary, even though we've evolved to move throughout the day. Get in steps and some natural movement where you can—there's no need to circle the parking lot at the grocery store, at work, or while running errands to park as close to the building as humanly possible.

Recent research published in the *American Journal of Public Health* looked at how a reminder note to start one habit can lead to other healthy practices, such as taking the stairs. When a sign was posted to "Take the Stairs" at the bottom of a stairwell, more people did. Use this in your own life with a note on your dashboard, on your bathroom mirror, on your fridge, or anywhere else you need it.

Install a browser extension or app to remind you to get up, stand, move, or stretch every hour.

Centenarians in the blue zones areas live in environments that nudge them to move naturally every twenty minutes, rather than separating fitness into a different part of their day. Activity is built into their lifestyles subconsciously. You can install a free app like StretchClock to be reminded to get up during your workday, and even to get suggested stretches to practice right next to your desk.

Take the bus or public transportation to work or to run an errand at least once.

The American Heart Association's research has found that people who regularly take public transit are 44 percent less likely to be overweight, 27 percent less likely to have high blood pressure, and 34 percent less likely to have diabetes, compared to people who drive.

Plan a walking meeting at work.

Walking meetings are a great way to keep you and your co-workers more active—and when weather permits, getting some sunshine and fresh air helps relieve stress. This effect is multiplied when you're walking in a group, since you're more likely to stick to a walking regimen.

Some companies actually make it a policy to prioritize walking meetings over sitting ones. Your workplace can also remove chairs and raise the table for a "standing" meeting room. I've seen other workplaces that have created walking paths on work grounds or walking route maps to the neighborhood around the office building. As with everything else in this book, if you can help make it easy for yourself and co-workers, they (and you) are more likely to do it.

But, here's the best part. In addition to stress management, a walking meeting can help boost creativity in your team. A recent survey by *Harvard Business Review* showed that walking team members say they are more creative.

Bringing a group of co-workers together can also engage employees who otherwise might not get involved. In one study done by Wellness & Prevention, Inc. at Johnson & Johnson, walking meeting groups reported that they felt more energized and more invested in their colleagues and organization. Management and employee barriers can also be lowered during a walking meeting.

Why Record What You Eat?

One of the things we know about blue zones populations is that their calorie intake is limited. *Hara hachi bu* is an Okinawan phrase that encourages Okinawans to stop eating when they are 80 percent full. Other cultures fast regularly for religious reasons.

Keeping a food diary can help you lose weight faster, and help you find and keep your ideal weight. Instead of mindlessly eating throughout the day as most of us do, it will help you understand what your true eating habits are. In one study of over 1,700 subjects published in the *American Journal of Preventive Medicine,* people who kept daily logs of what they ate lost twice the amount of weight as those who didn't. Another recent study published in *Obesity: The Journal of the Obesity Society* shows that an accurate, daily food diary is one of the most effective weight loss habits that can be practiced.

For the best results, record what you eat immediately after eating. The more accurate your information, the more you'll learn about yourself.

IKARIAN
LONGEVITY STEW

Total cook time: 1 hour, 15 minutes | Makes 4 servings

. . . .

INGREDIENTS

½ cup extra virgin olive oil, divided

1 large red onion, finely chopped

4 garlic cloves, finely chopped

1 fennel bulb, chopped

1 cup (8 ounces) dried black-eyed peas or 15 ounces canned*

1 large, firm ripe tomato, finely chopped

2 teaspoons tomato paste, diluted in ¼ cup water

2 bay leaves

1 bunch dill, finely chopped

Salt to taste

STEPS

1. Heat ¼ cup of the olive oil over medium heat and add the onion, garlic, and fennel bulb. Cook, stirring occasionally, until soft, about 12 minutes. Add the black-eyed peas and toss to coat in the oil.

2. Add the tomato, tomato paste, and enough water to cover the beans by about 1 inch. Add the bay leaves. Bring to a boil, reduce the heat, and simmer until the black-eyed peas are about halfway cooked. Check after 40 minutes, but cooking may take over an hour.

3. Add the chopped dill and season with salt.

4. Continue cooking until the black-eyed peas are tender. Remove the bay leaves, stir in the remaining olive oil, and serve.

*For dried peas, cover with water, bring to a boil, boil for 1 minute, remove from the heat, cover, and let sit for 1 hour. Drain, rinse, and use.

SWEET POTATO BLACK BEAN BURGER

Total cook time: 35 minutes | Makes 4 servings

INGREDIENTS

The Patty

1½ cups rolled oats

1 cup peeled, cooked, and mashed sweet potato

1 cup cooked, mashed black beans

½ teaspoon salt

2 teaspoons onion powder

1 teaspoon ground cumin

1 teaspoon smoked paprika

½ teaspoon black pepper

½ teaspoon chipotle powder (optional)

Oil for cooking

The Sauce

¼ cup toasted pepitas

½ cup good-quality salsa verde

The Toppings

1 avocado

½ cup loosely packed sliced kale

Pickled or thinly sliced raw red onion*

4 whole wheat burger buns

STEPS

1. To make the patties, pulse the rolled oats in a food processor until coarsely ground and set aside.

2. Combine the sweet potato, black beans, salt, and spices; then incorporate the ground oats. Let this sit for about 5 minutes so the flavors can marry.

3. Form the mixture into 4 patties.

4. In a skillet, heat a thin layer of oil over medium heat. Add the patties and fry on both sides until crisped, about 4 minutes per side.

5. To make the sauce: Puree the pepitas and salsa verde in a food processor or blender and set aside.

6. Build your burger: Mash the avocado and spread it on the bottom half of a bun. Then, add your patty and top with the pepita sauce. Finish off the burger with kale and red onion, then add the top half of the bun.

*To pickle red onions, submerge thin slices in white vinegar with a generous pinch of salt and let sit for at least 6 hours.

DAN'S LONGEVITY
DAL PALAK

Total cook time: 35 minutes | Makes 4 servings

. . . .

INGREDIENTS

1 teaspoon garam masala

1 teaspoon turmeric

1 teaspoon salt

1 onion, chopped

4 to 5 cloves garlic, separated, chopped finely

1-inch piece of ginger root, peeled and chopped

1 teaspoon red pepper flakes

⅓ cup oil

1 can (15 ounces) chopped tomatoes

1 cup lentils

2½ cups water

1 cup spinach leaves

Salt to taste

STEPS

1. Sauté the garam masala, turmeric, salt, onion, garlic, ginger, and red pepper flakes in the oil until the onions are clear.

2. Add the tomatoes, lentils, and water; simmer for 30 minutes.

3. Add the spinach and stir until wilted. Season with salt to taste.

4. Serve over rice or with naan.

ADVENTIST HAYSTACKS

Total cook time: 15 minutes | Makes 6 servings

INGREDIENTS

2 cups lightly salted or low-sodium tortilla chips (use blue corn chips for a nice presentation)

2 cups shredded romaine lettuce

1 avocado, chopped

1 Roma tomato, chopped

½ cup corn kernels

1 cup cooked dried black beans or 8-ounce can (drained and rinsed if using canned)*

1 cup good-quality salsa

Suggested Toppings

Sliced pickled jalapeños

2 to 3 green onions, sliced

Chopped cilantro (optional)

Cashew cream drizzle (optional)

½ cup meatless crumbles (optional)

STEPS

1. If assembling as a completed dish, on a large platter spread a layer of tortilla chips.

2. Then add a layer of lettuce and the chopped vegetables, followed by a layer of beans, then the salsa.

3. Add all the toppings, then drizzle with cashew cream and add a sprinkle of meatless crumbles, if desired.

4. Following this assembly order keeps the chips from getting soggy, allowing you to make this dish ahead of time.

NOTE: Feel free to get creative. Play with adding olives, cucumbers, zucchini, roasted red peppers, pepitas, or whatever other veggies you have on hand to create your own version of a haystack, adding these between the lettuce and bean layers. You can also alter the flavor by changing up the salsa you use as the dressing.

OKINAWAN CREAM OF MUSHROOM SOUP

Total cook time: 20 minutes | Makes 4 servings

INGREDIENTS

1 small onion or ¾ cup leeks, chopped

1 tablespoon vegetable oil

1 teaspoon salt

1½ cups shiitake mushrooms (or use ½ cup each of shiitake, enoki, and shimeji mushrooms)

1 teaspoon grated ginger

2 cups plain soy milk

1 bay leaf

1 tablespoon miso paste

STEPS

1. In a large pot, stir-fry the onion in the vegetable oil with a dash of salt until soft, 5 to 6 minutes.

2. Add the mushrooms and continue sautéing until soft.

3. Add the ginger, soy milk, and bay leaf and bring to a simmer. Simmer for 3 minutes.

4. Turn off the heat, remove the bay leaf, and stir in the miso before serving.

PUMPKIN PANCAKES

Total cook time: 10 minutes | Makes 4 servings

INGREDIENTS

1 cup oat flour (store-bought or make by blending quick oats)

1 teaspoon cinnamon

½ tablespoon baking powder

¼ cup vanilla soy or almond milk

½ cup pumpkin puree

¼ cup applesauce

1 tablespoon apple cider vinegar

1½ tablespoons honey

Oil for greasing the pan

STEPS

1. In a large bowl, mix all the dry ingredients together.

2. Add the wet ingredients and mix until combined. Let the batter sit for 3 to 4 minutes to thicken.

3. Heat a nonstick pan over medium heat. Once the pan is hot, reduce the heat to medium-low. Oil the pan lightly and gently pour spoonfuls of batter into the circular size you want.

4. Flip after 1 to 2 minutes, or when small bubbles begin to form, and cook the other sides another 1 to 2 minutes.

5. Repeat until the batter is used up.

The Blue Zones Challenge
WEEK 3

Week 3 Activities

- Eat at least three Blue Zones meals this week.
- Join a new social group (church, school club, local organization, team sport).
- Walk with your group or buddy at least once.
- Volunteer to be an organ donor (on your driver's license).
- Volunteer for a new organization.
- Call, text, or email one friend or family member you haven't connected with recently.
- Plan a vacation or some time off work.
- Start a meditation practice (p. 162).
- Put a lavender plant in your bedroom (p. 161).
- Write a thank-you note (p. 161).
- Schedule a weekly get-together with friends (Friday happy hour, workout session, book club, game night).

WEEKLY BONUS POINTS

ACTIVITY	POINTS
Walked or ate with my *moai* or Blue Zones buddy (3 points each time)	
Volunteered for at least 30 minutes (3 points each time)	
Tried new Blue Zones recipes (goal = 3 recipes) (1 for each recipe)	
Completed other Blue Zones activities this week (2 for each activity)	
Spent at least 30 minutes engaged in a hobby or passion (1 point each time)	

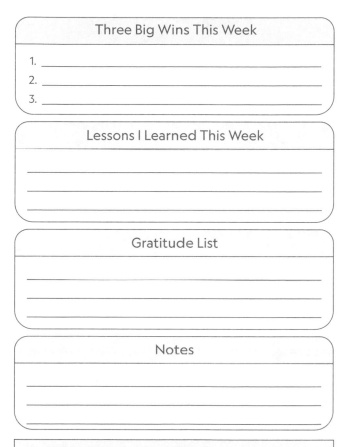

Three Big Wins This Week

1. _____
2. _____
3. _____

Lessons I Learned This Week

_____
_____
_____

Gratitude List

_____
_____
_____

Notes

_____
_____
_____

The Blue Zones Challenge
DAILY CHECK-IN

Track your progress every day to see how you're reshaping your environment, the spaces in which you live, your health, and your happiness. Each of the daily worksheets on the following pages will help you record the activities, foods, and steps you're taking toward a Blue Zones lifestyle. Keep track of how you're doing with the daily scorecard—you should improve each day and week.

DAY 8 SCORECARD

ACTIVITY	POINTS
Ate 100% whole-food, plant-based diet today (5 points)	
Ate a cup of beans today (3 points)	
Consumed all meals / calories within 10-hour window (2 points)	
Walked or did some other physical activity at least 30 minutes today (can be multiple walks) (2 points)	
Screen time less than 1 hour (outside work / school) (2 points)	
Recorded my weight (1 point)	
Recorded what I ate (1 point)	
Servings of poultry, pork, beef, lamb (-1 per serving)	
Servings of cow's milk products (milk, cheese, etc.) (-1 per serving)	
Servings of processed foods (packaged cookies, candies, chips, etc.) (-1 per serving)	
Servings of sweetened beverages (soda, fruit drinks, sport drinks) (-1 per serving)	
DAILY SCORE:	

DAILY TARGET = 12 POINTS A DAY

DAY 9 SCORECARD

ACTIVITY	POINTS
Ate 100% whole-food, plant-based diet today (5 points)	
Ate a cup of beans today (3 points)	
Consumed all meals / calories within 10-hour window (2 points)	
Walked or did some other physical activity at least 30 minutes today (can be multiple walks) (2 points)	
Screen time less than 1 hour (outside work / school) (2 points)	
Recorded my weight (1 point)	
Recorded what I ate (1 point)	
Servings of poultry, pork, beef, lamb (-1 per serving)	
Servings of cow's milk products (milk, cheese, etc.) (-1 per serving)	
Servings of processed foods (packaged cookies, candies, chips, etc.) (-1 per serving)	
Servings of sweetened beverages (soda, fruit drinks, sport drinks) (-1 per serving)	
DAILY SCORE:	

DAILY TARGET = 12 POINTS A DAY

DAY 10 SCORECARD

ACTIVITY	POINTS
Ate 100% whole-food, plant-based diet today (5 points)	
Ate a cup of beans today (3 points)	
Consumed all meals / calories within 10-hour window (2 points)	
Walked or did some other physical activity at least 30 minutes today (can be multiple walks) (2 points)	
Screen time less than 1 hour (outside work / school) (2 points)	
Recorded my weight (1 point)	
Recorded what I ate (1 point)	
Servings of poultry, pork, beef, lamb (-1 per serving)	
Servings of cow's milk products (milk, cheese, etc.) (-1 per serving)	
Servings of processed foods (packaged cookies, candies, chips, etc.) (-1 per serving)	
Servings of sweetened beverages (soda, fruit drinks, sport drinks) (-1 per serving)	
DAILY SCORE:	

DAILY TARGET = 12 POINTS A DAY

DAY 11 SCORECARD

ACTIVITY	POINTS
Ate 100% whole-food, plant-based diet today (5 points)	
Ate a cup of beans today (3 points)	
Consumed all meals / calories within 10-hour window (2 points)	
Walked or did some other physical activity at least 30 minutes today (can be multiple walks) (2 points)	
Screen time less than 1 hour (outside work / school) (2 points)	
Recorded my weight (1 point)	
Recorded what I ate (1 point)	
Servings of poultry, pork, beef, lamb (-1 per serving)	
Servings of cow's milk products (milk, cheese, etc.) (-1 per serving)	
Servings of processed foods (packaged cookies, candies, chips, etc.) (-1 per serving)	
Servings of sweetened beverages (soda, fruit drinks, sport drinks) (-1 per serving)	
DAILY SCORE:	

DAILY TARGET = 12 POINTS A DAY

DAY 12 SCORECARD

ACTIVITY	POINTS
Ate 100% whole-food, plant-based diet today (5 points)	
Ate a cup of beans today (3 points)	
Consumed all meals / calories within 10-hour window (2 points)	
Walked or did some other physical activity at least 30 minutes today (can be multiple walks) (2 points)	
Screen time less than 1 hour (outside work / school) (2 points)	
Recorded my weight (1 point)	
Recorded what I ate (1 point)	
Servings of poultry, pork, beef, lamb (-1 per serving)	
Servings of cow's milk products (milk, cheese, etc.) (-1 per serving)	
Servings of processed foods (packaged cookies, candies, chips, etc.) (-1 per serving)	
Servings of sweetened beverages (soda, fruit drinks, sport drinks) (-1 per serving)	
DAILY SCORE:	

DAILY TARGET = 12 POINTS A DAY

DAY 13 SCORECARD

ACTIVITY	POINTS
Ate 100% whole-food, plant-based diet today (5 points)	
Ate a cup of beans today (3 points)	
Consumed all meals / calories within 10-hour window (2 points)	
Walked or did some other physical activity at least 30 minutes today (can be multiple walks) (2 points)	
Screen time less than 1 hour (outside work / school) (2 points)	
Recorded my weight (1 point)	
Recorded what I ate (1 point)	
Servings of poultry, pork, beef, lamb (-1 per serving)	
Servings of cow's milk products (milk, cheese, etc.) (-1 per serving)	
Servings of processed foods (packaged cookies, candies, chips, etc.) (-1 per serving)	
Servings of sweetened beverages (soda, fruit drinks, sport drinks) (-1 per serving)	
DAILY SCORE:	

DAILY TARGET = 12 POINTS A DAY

DAY 14 SCORECARD

ACTIVITY	POINTS
Ate 100% whole-food, plant-based diet today (5 points)	
Ate a cup of beans today (3 points)	
Consumed all meals / calories within 10-hour window (2 points)	
Walked or did some other physical activity at least 30 minutes today (can be multiple walks) (2 points)	
Screen time less than 1 hour (outside work / school) (2 points)	
Recorded my weight (1 point)	
Recorded what I ate (1 point)	
Servings of poultry, pork, beef, lamb (-1 per serving)	
Servings of cow's milk products (milk, cheese, etc.) (-1 per serving)	
Servings of processed foods (packaged cookies, candies, chips, etc.) (-1 per serving)	
Servings of sweetened beverages (soda, fruit drinks, sport drinks) (-1 per serving)	
DAILY SCORE:	

DAILY TARGET = 12 POINTS A DAY

WEEKLY SCORE BOX

Weekly Score = Daily Totals +
Weekly Bonus Points

Week 1: _____ Week 2: _____ Week 3: _____

Target: 400 points for the whole month

Tips and Tricks
. . . .

Write a thank-you note to a co-worker or friend.

Research published in *Psychological Science* says that when people express their gratitude, it improves both their own happiness and the well-being and happiness of the person they are thanking.

Put a lavender plant in your bedroom.

The smell is calming and can help induce sleep.

Volunteer to be an organ donor (on your driver's license).

"If you want to do a random act of kindness, there isn't a more powerful few minutes than signing to be an organ donor. You never have to lift a finger. It is the laziest, most excellent good deed that you can do that will give you a happiness boost." —Gretchen Rubin, author of *The Happiness Project*

Join a new social group (church, school club, local group, volunteer opportunity, etc.).

This can be a new group at your temple, church, or other faith-based community; a new club at your school; or a local group like Meetup. Our friends and social groups shape our lives (and our waistlines).

Start a meditation practice.

Practiced since ancient times, and often in conjunction with religious traditions, meditation has been taken up by the masses. A National Health Interview Survey showed that meditation practice among adults tripled between 2012 and 2017. We also know that the blue zones share a "downshift" habit—a time when the day's stressors can be released.

There are many different meditation practices. They all typically involve a quiet, comfortable place to relax, a comfortable position (either sitting or lying down) that promotes meditation, focused attention, and letting distractions go as they come up. There are forms of "walking meditation" as well, but they have not been studied as thoroughly. Either way, setting aside as little as 15 minutes a day to "downshift" can benefit you in many ways.

Emotional benefits include:
- Increased self-awareness, which may also help you find a purpose, or *ikigai*—another blue zones shared trait
- Help in reducing negative emotions that contribute to stress
- Development of skills to manage stress
- Increased creativity
- Reduced symptoms of anxiety and depression

Since meditation has been shown to reverse the stress response, physical benefits include:
- Lowered blood pressure
- Reduced inflammation
- Support for smoking cessation programs
- Reduced symptoms of ulcerative colitis and irritable bowel syndrome
- Treatment for chronic insomnia

To get started on your own, set yourself up for success:
1. Subscribe to a free meditation app or enroll in a series of meditation classes.
2. Set up a meditation nook in a corner or room of your house so you have a place to meditate. It should be a quiet place with a cushion you can sit on, decorated with the things that inspire you to downshift. Seeing this setup will be a visual reminder for you to meditate.

Screen Time

Aim for no more than one hour of additional screen time daily (including Netflix, TV shows, news).

Americans spend an average of over six hours a day staring at screens—watching, scrolling, working, studying. It can easily get in the way of the face-to-face interactions so important to living the Blue Zones life.

Also, people who watch too much TV are more likely to be overweight. TV watching actually lowers metabolism, makes us less active, and encourages us via commercials to eat junk food. Research shows that kids with a TV in their bedroom are 18 percent more likely to be (or become) obese and have lower grades; in addition, the happiest people watch only 30 to 60 minutes of TV per day.

Stress and Downshifting

Stress is part of the human condition. People in blue zones suffer the same stresses that others do. However, the people living in blue zones have daily rituals that reduce their stress and reverse the inflammation associated with it. The rituals vary and include activities such as prayer, ancestor veneration, napping, and happy hour. Even other parts of the Blue Zones lifestyle, including a strong community of family and friends, a healthy diet, and regular natural movement, contribute to stress reduction and better mental well-being.

POTATO LEEK SOUP

Total cook time: 45 minutes | Makes 4 servings

INGREDIENTS

2 medium leeks, cut into ¼-inch slices

1 clove garlic, minced

1 tablespoon olive oil

2 medium potatoes (Yukon Gold work best), cubed

2 cups veggie chicken-flavor broth or vegetable broth

1 cup unflavored soy milk

Salt and pepper to taste

Chopped scallions or chives for garnish (optional)

STEPS

1. In a large soup pot, sauté the leeks and garlic in the olive oil until fragrant, about 8 minutes.

2. Add the potatoes and broth, bring to a simmer, and cook for 30 minutes.

3. In batches, very briefly process the soup mixture in a blender (no more than half full) with the soy milk.

4. Return the soup to the pot and cook over medium heat until heated through.

5. Season with salt and pepper to taste and serve garnished with chives or scallions, if using.

IKARIAN STUFFED EGGPLANT (IMAM BAYILDI)

Total cook time: 1 hour | Makes 4 servings

INGREDIENTS

5 medium eggplants, ends cut off, scored deeply four times lengthwise

1¼ cups extra-virgin olive oil, divided

1 cup parsley, chopped

2 large tomatoes, diced

2 onions, diced

4 cloves garlic, sliced in thirds

1 bell pepper (green, red, or yellow), diced

1 potato, peeled and thinly sliced

Salt and pepper, to taste

STEPS

1. In a large pan, sauté the eggplants over medium-high heat in ¼ cup of the olive oil for about 10 minutes, rotating often.

2. While the eggplants cook, in a medium bowl, mix together the parsley, tomatoes, onions, garlic, bell pepper, and the remaining 1 cup olive oil as your stuffing mixture.

3. In a separate pan, sauté the stuffing for 6 to 8 minutes, or until the onions are tender.

4. Add the stuffing mix on top of the eggplants. Place potatoes around the eggplants in the pan.

5. Cook over low heat for about 30 minutes, checking the pan for any cooking liquid and basting with it if needed.

ADVENTIST BROWN RICE SALAD

Total cook time: 10 minutes | Makes 2 servings

INGREDIENTS

1/8 teaspoon turmeric

1/4 teaspoon salt

1 tablespoon lemon juice

2 teaspoons olive oil

2 Persian cucumbers, sliced or diced

1/2 red bell pepper, cored and sliced or diced

3 black pitted olives, diced

2 teaspoons pine nuts (or substitute other chopped nuts)

1 tablespoon fresh parsley, minced

1 cup cooked brown rice

STEPS

1. In a large bowl, whisk together the turmeric, salt, lemon juice, and olive oil.

2. Add all the other ingredients except for rice to the bowl and mix well with the dressing until coated.

3. Add the rice and toss to combine well. If using just-cooked rice, chill the salad in refrigerator for 1 to 2 hours before serving.

OKINAWA THREE-MINUTE NOODLES

Total cook time: 15 minutes | Makes 4 servings

INGREDIENTS

1 pound somen noodles

2 tablespoons sesame oil, divided

8 ounces firm tofu, drained and cut into 1-inch chunks

¼ cup chopped garlic chives (or scallions)

Soy sauce, to taste

STEPS

1. Cook the noodles according to package directions, for 2 to 3 minutes.

2. Drain and mix the noodles with 1 tablespoon of the sesame oil so they don't stick together.

3. In a large sauté pan, heat the remaining 1 tablespoon sesame oil over medium-high heat, add the tofu, and cook until it's browned, 3 to 4 minutes per side.

4. Add the chives and the somen noodles to the pan and mix well.

5. Season to taste with a splash or two of soy sauce.

ROASTED POTATOES AND GREEN BEANS WITH MUSTARD DRIZZLE

Total cook time: 45 minutes | Makes 4 servings

INGREDIENTS

Potatoes and Green Beans

½ pound fingerling potatoes

3 garlic cloves

3 tablespoons chopped fresh parsley or other herbs

1½ tablespoons extra-virgin olive oil

½ cup cooked chickpeas (or canned, drained and rinsed), patted dry with a paper towel

½ pound green beans

Mustard Drizzle

1 tablespoon Dijon mustard

1½ tablespoons extra-virgin olive oil

1 tablespoon white wine vinegar

2 teaspoons honey

Salt and pepper, to taste

STEPS

1. Heat the oven to 425 degrees F.

2. In a large mixing bowl, toss the potatoes with the garlic, herbs, and olive oil.

3. Place the mixture in a single layer on a roasting pan and roast in the oven for 25 minutes, stirring once or twice.

4. When the potatoes are tender and starting to brown, add the chickpeas and green beans to the pan and roast for another 10 minutes.

5. Meanwhile, in a small bowl whisk together the mustard, olive oil, vinegar, and honey to form an emulsified dressing. Season with salt and pepper to taste.

6. Transfer the roasted vegetables and beans to a platter and drizzle with the mustard dressing. Serve warm.

The Blue Zones Challenge
WEEK 4

Week 4 Activities

- Review your Purpose Statement, and reflect on how you are living your purpose each day.
- Eat at least three Blue Zones meals this week.
- Walk with your group or buddy at least once.
- Designate a space in your home for quiet time, meditation, or prayer (p. 182).
- Enroll in an automatic savings or investment plan.
- Get blackout shades or an eye mask to block out light when you sleep (p. 181).
- Volunteer for a new group or organization (p. 180).
- Declutter your house.
- Practice listening to someone with great attention.
- Enjoy a Japanese or Costa Rican breakfast (p. 182).
- Start a container or outdoor garden (p. 181).
- Consider adopting a dog or a cat.

WEEKLY BONUS POINTS

ACTIVITY	POINTS
Walked or ate with my *moai* or Blue Zones buddy (3 points each time)	
Volunteered for at least 30 minutes (3 points each time)	
Tried new Blue Zones recipes (goal = 3 recipes) (1 for each recipe)	
Completed other Blue Zones activities this week (2 for each activity)	
Spent at least 30 minutes engaged in a hobby or passion (1 point each time)	

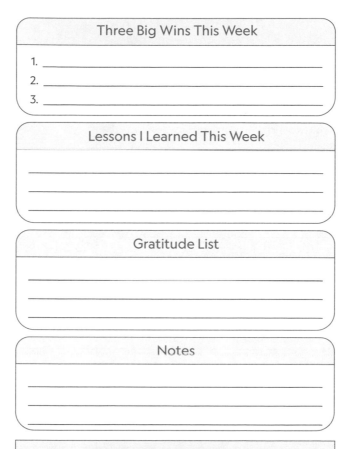

Three Big Wins This Week

1. _____
2. _____
3. _____

Lessons I Learned This Week

_____

_____

_____

Gratitude List

_____

_____

_____

Notes

_____

_____

_____

The Blue Zones Challenge
DAILY CHECK-IN

Track your progress every day to see how you're reshaping your environment, the spaces in which you live, your health, and your happiness. Each of the daily worksheets on the following pages will help you record the activities, foods, and steps you're taking toward a Blue Zones lifestyle. Keep track of how you're doing with the daily scorecard—you should improve each day and week.

DAY 15 SCORECARD

ACTIVITY	POINTS
Ate 100% whole-food, plant-based diet today (5 points)	
Ate a cup of beans today (3 points)	
Consumed all meals / calories within 10-hour window (2 points)	
Walked or did some other physical activity at least 30 minutes today (can be multiple walks) (2 points)	
Screen time less than 1 hour (outside work / school) (2 points)	
Recorded my weight (1 point)	
Recorded what I ate (1 point)	
Servings of poultry, pork, beef, lamb (-1 per serving)	
Servings of cow's milk products (milk, cheese, etc.) (-1 per serving)	
Servings of processed foods (packaged cookies, candies, chips, etc.) (-1 per serving)	
Servings of sweetened beverages (soda, fruit drinks, sport drinks) (-1 per serving)	
DAILY SCORE:	

DAILY TARGET = 12 POINTS A DAY

DAY 16 SCORECARD

ACTIVITY	POINTS
Ate 100% whole-food, plant-based diet today (5 points)	
Ate a cup of beans today (3 points)	
Consumed all meals / calories within 10-hour window (2 points)	
Walked or did some other physical activity at least 30 minutes today (can be multiple walks) (2 points)	
Screen time less than 1 hour (outside work / school) (2 points)	
Recorded my weight (1 point)	
Recorded what I ate (1 point)	
Servings of poultry, pork, beef, lamb (-1 per serving)	
Servings of cow's milk products (milk, cheese, etc.) (-1 per serving)	
Servings of processed foods (packaged cookies, candies, chips, etc.) (-1 per serving)	
Servings of sweetened beverages (soda, fruit drinks, sport drinks) (-1 per serving)	
DAILY SCORE:	

DAILY TARGET = 12 POINTS A DAY

DAY 17 SCORECARD

ACTIVITY	POINTS
Ate 100% whole-food, plant-based diet today (5 points)	
Ate a cup of beans today (3 points)	
Consumed all meals / calories within 10-hour window (2 points)	
Walked or did some other physical activity at least 30 minutes today (can be multiple walks) (2 points)	
Screen time less than 1 hour (outside work / school) (2 points)	
Recorded my weight (1 point)	
Recorded what I ate (1 point)	
Servings of poultry, pork, beef, lamb (-1 per serving)	
Servings of cow's milk products (milk, cheese, etc.) (-1 per serving)	
Servings of processed foods (packaged cookies, candies, chips, etc.) (-1 per serving)	
Servings of sweetened beverages (soda, fruit drinks, sport drinks) (-1 per serving)	
DAILY SCORE:	

DAILY TARGET = 12 POINTS A DAY

DAY 18 SCORECARD

ACTIVITY	POINTS
Ate 100% whole-food, plant-based diet today (5 points)	
Ate a cup of beans today (3 points)	
Consumed all meals / calories within 10-hour window (2 points)	
Walked or did some other physical activity at least 30 minutes today (can be multiple walks) (2 points)	
Screen time less than 1 hour (outside work / school) (2 points)	
Recorded my weight (1 point)	
Recorded what I ate (1 point)	
Servings of poultry, pork, beef, lamb (-1 per serving)	
Servings of cow's milk products (milk, cheese, etc.) (-1 per serving)	
Servings of processed foods (packaged cookies, candies, chips, etc.) (-1 per serving)	
Servings of sweetened beverages (soda, fruit drinks, sport drinks) (-1 per serving)	
DAILY SCORE:	

DAILY TARGET = 12 POINTS A DAY

DAY 19 SCORECARD

ACTIVITY	POINTS
Ate 100% whole-food, plant-based diet today (5 points)	
Ate a cup of beans today (3 points)	
Consumed all meals / calories within 10-hour window (2 points)	
Walked or did some other physical activity at least 30 minutes today (can be multiple walks) (2 points)	
Screen time less than 1 hour (outside work / school) (2 points)	
Recorded my weight (1 point)	
Recorded what I ate (1 point)	
Servings of poultry, pork, beef, lamb (-1 per serving)	
Servings of cow's milk products (milk, cheese, etc.) (-1 per serving)	
Servings of processed foods (packaged cookies, candies, chips, etc.) (-1 per serving)	
Servings of sweetened beverages (soda, fruit drinks, sport drinks) (-1 per serving)	
DAILY SCORE:	

DAILY TARGET = 12 POINTS A DAY

DAY 20 SCORECARD

ACTIVITY	POINTS
Ate 100% whole-food, plant-based diet today (5 points)	
Ate a cup of beans today (3 points)	
Consumed all meals / calories within 10-hour window (2 points)	
Walked or did some other physical activity at least 30 minutes today (can be multiple walks) (2 points)	
Screen time less than 1 hour (outside work / school) (2 points)	
Recorded my weight (1 point)	
Recorded what I ate (1 point)	
Servings of poultry, pork, beef, lamb (-1 per serving)	
Servings of cow's milk products (milk, cheese, etc.) (-1 per serving)	
Servings of processed foods (packaged cookies, candies, chips, etc.) (-1 per serving)	
Servings of sweetened beverages (soda, fruit drinks, sport drinks) (-1 per serving)	
DAILY SCORE:	

DAILY TARGET = 12 POINTS A DAY

DAY 21 SCORECARD

ACTIVITY	POINTS
Ate 100% whole-food, plant-based diet today (5 points)	
Ate a cup of beans today (3 points)	
Consumed all meals / calories within 10-hour window (2 points)	
Walked or did some other physical activity at least 30 minutes today (can be multiple walks) (2 points)	
Screen time less than 1 hour (outside work / school) (2 points)	
Recorded my weight (1 point)	
Recorded what I ate (1 point)	
Servings of poultry, pork, beef, lamb (-1 per serving)	
Servings of cow's milk products (milk, cheese, etc.) (-1 per serving)	
Servings of processed foods (packaged cookies, candies, chips, etc.) (-1 per serving)	
Servings of sweetened beverages (soda, fruit drinks, sport drinks) (-1 per serving)	
DAILY SCORE:	

DAILY TARGET = 12 POINTS A DAY

WEEKLY SCORE BOX

Week 1: _____

Week 2: _____

Week 3: _____

Week 4: _____

TOTAL: _____

Target: 400 points for the whole month

MADE IT TO 400 POINTS?

People who make it to 400 points this month should see their life expectancy jump. And the deeper you go into the Blue Zones lifestyle, the better you'll feel.

Made it to 400 points? Head to bluezones.com/400Club to add your name to the list of challenge finishers!

Tips and Tricks

. . . .

Volunteer for a new group or organization.

Altruism stimulates the same neural pathways as sugar and cocaine. But unlike drugs, volunteering is a healthy addiction. People who volunteer tend to lose weight, have lower rates of heart disease, and report higher levels of happiness. Volunteering also opens up opportunities to meet like-minded people with the same values. Decide what you do best and volunteer your time.

If you're having a hard time figuring out where to volunteer:

1. Refer to the purpose exercise (see page 79) to recall your purpose and Purpose Statement.

2. Talk to your *moai* or Blue Zones buddy to discuss an organization you might all want to join and volunteer together.

3. Start with a Google search or look for organizations on sites like VolunteerMatch.

4. Call or email organizations that most interest you. Ask if they have an initiation period or some sort of training to see if it's the right fit for you. If you don't have a positive experience the first time you go, then you won't want to go back. Remember: For it to be sustainable, it must be an experience that you like.

5. Ask about opportunities to socialize or connect

with other volunteers. Remember: This could be a good place for you to build your social circle with like-minded people.

6. Ask how the organization recognizes volunteers. The best ones have volunteer socials or recognition events.

Start a container or outdoor garden.

In all blue zones, people continue to garden even into their 90s and 100s. Gardening is the epitome of a blue zones activity because it's sort of a nudge: You plant the seeds and you're going to be nudged in the next three to four months to water the plants, weed them, harvest them. And when you're done, you're going to eat an organic vegetable, which you presumably like because you planted it. So you're moving naturally while you're outside enjoying the healing power of the sun and nature and fresh air.

Get blackout shades or an eye mask to block out light when you sleep.

Centenarians in the blue zones areas of the world sleep seven to eight hours every night and have daily routines to help them downshift. (See page 184 for more on sleep.)

Consider adopting a dog or a cat.

If you feel ready to be a responsible pet owner, pets make for great companions, and dogs in particular encourage you to walk or run. Researchers have found that if you own a dog, you get more than five hours of exercise a week without a lot of added effort. In fact, studies have shown that dog owners have lower rates of health problems compared to those who don't own a dog.

Designate a space in your home for quiet time, meditation, or prayer.

Create space in your home, even if it's just a corner, where you can relax without distraction. Just as a dedicated, distraction-free workspace can improve focus while you're working, a dedicated, distraction-free space can improve your downshift practices, even if it's just reading a book or listening to music.

Enjoy a Japanese or Costa Rican breakfast.

Breakfast in the blue zones looks vastly different from the standard American breakfast of eggs and bacon. Beans are a common breakfast staple in Costa Rica, while miso soup and rice are popular in Okinawa. In Loma Linda, centenarians often eat a hearty breakfast of oatmeal or a somewhat nontraditional tofu scramble.

In most blue zones regions, breakfast doesn't look that different from other meals of the day. Retraining yourself to enjoy soup and bread or even a hearty salad and sandwich in the morning might take some getting used to, but it's an easy way to simplify your cooking routine as well as cutting out American breakfast favorites that are most often heavy in fat and sugar.

Put together a hearty meal using any of the four Blue Zones breakfast basics: cooked whole grains, fruit and veggie smoothies, and beans. See page 123 for a breakfast recipe that uses whole grains.

Purpose and Passion

People in the blue zones don't wake up feeling rudderless. They're driven by their life's meaning and purpose. They're investing in family, keeping their minds engaged, and keeping daily rituals to downshift and reduce stress.

In the blue zones, people have vocabulary for purpose, and the idea of "why I wake up in the morning" is an integral part of their culture. More important, we think that this strong sense of purpose may in fact reduce their chances of suffering from Alzheimer's disease, arthritis, and stroke. A study from the National Institute on Aging found that people who could articulate their sense of purpose were living up to seven years longer.

Another study, funded by the National Institutes of Health, that looked at the correlation between having a sense of purpose and longevity found that healthy people between the ages of 65 and 92 who expressed having clear goals or purpose lived longer and lived better than those who did not. This is because individuals who understand what brings them joy and happiness tend to have what we like to call the right outlook. They are engulfed in activities and communities that allow them to immerse themselves in a rewarding and gratifying environment.

Sleep

One of the benefits of healthy sleep patterns is improved cognition and mood; when we get enough sleep, we're able to think and process information better, and our general mood is more positive. We know, for example, that chronic sleep disruption makes you more prone to depression. At the same time, chronic depression can contribute to sleep deprivation—a downward spiral, to say the least.

Other benefits (and problems if you're not getting enough sleep) can be seen in these areas:
- Heart health: When you're sleeping, your blood pressure decreases. This gives your heart and blood vessels time to rest and repair. Chronic high blood pressure contributes to stroke risk and heart disease.

- Blood sugar: Deep sleep induces a drop in blood sugar levels. With better blood sugar regulation, you're less likely to develop type 2 diabetes.
- Healthy weight: Key hormones that control appetite are well regulated when you're getting enough sleep. When you're not, the balance of these hormones (leptin and ghrelin) is disrupted, which makes you more prone to eat junk and eat too much.
- Immune health: When you're sleeping well, your immune system is well rested and ready to launch an attack when you encounter harmful bacteria or a virus. If you're not sleeping well, your immune system is tired too and may not be equipped to fight off an attack quickly or with much effect. You might also find yourself getting sick more often.

If you're experiencing sleep problems, make sure you're eating well, moving enough, and taking time to relax every day. Setting up a regular sleep time, as well as a bedtime routine, can also help. Pay special attention to creating an environment in your home where getting a good night's sleep is easy.

Week 4 Check-In
· ·

You're done with the first four weeks of the rest of your Blue Zones life!

At the end of your four weeks, many positive changes have likely happened. You might feel great, are better rested, have maybe lost weight, feel happier, are better connected to your friends and family. But even if you have just improved in a couple of those areas of your life (not all), we think you'll be so happy about the changes that have worked that you will continue on for another four weeks. And another. And so on.

Continue using this planner to track your progress and your accomplishments. Check back in often and take stock of where you are.

Record and Reflect on Your Progress

Retest! Go back to the tests you took at the beginning of the challenge to see how far you've come in changing your habits, environment, and behavior. In each instance, you'll see a marked difference in your overall health, happiness, and well-being. Go ahead and record your metrics too—weight, BMI, cholesterol, etc.—so you can mark the noticeable changes in your health. Then reflect on the goals you've achieved and the goals you'd still like to work toward as you continue to live a Blue Zones life.

Record Your Results Here

True Vitality Test	
Week 1:	
Week 4:	

True Happiness Test	
Week 1:	
Week 4:	

Purpose Checkup	
Week 1:	
Week 4:	

Metrics Checkup	
Weight, Week 1:	
Weight, Week 4:	
BMI, Week 1:	
BMI, Week 4:	
Clothing Size, Week 1:	
Clothing Size, Week 4:	
Waist, Week 1:	
Waist, Week 4:	

How did your goals shift throughout the last four weeks? What goals did you achieve, and what goals are you still working toward?

_____

_____

_____

_____

Has your Purpose Statement changed at all? If so, how? Rewrite it here and post it where you can see it.

_____

_____

_____

How do you feel at the end of these first four weeks in terms of health, happiness, and your sense of purpose?

_____

_____

_____

What will motivate you to continue to practice a Blue Zones lifestyle throughout the rest of the year—and the rest of your life?

_____

_____

_____

_____

Celebrate Yourself

You've completed the first four weeks of the Blue Zones Challenge, and while you have a lifetime ahead of you, the hardest part is over. You've now set up the places you live, socialize, and work to provide a great environment to make the healthy choice the easy choice. You've expanded your social network to include healthy, like-minded friends who can be on this journey with you. And you're seeing results. Take this moment to celebrate the promise you made, and publicly declare you're going to continue following the Blue Zones lifestyle for years to come— hopefully well into your 90s and 100s.

Celebrate Online

Make it public. Share that you've completed your four-week challenge on Facebook, Twitter, or Instagram. You can post a before-and-after photo, an inspiring message, or an update on your progress—whatever feels most authentic and comfortable for you to share. Don't forget to proclaim your dedication to a Blue Zones life for the rest of your life. And include #bluezoneslife to share with the Blue Zones community and inspire others.

Celebrate With Your *Moai*

You couldn't have done this challenge alone—in fact, you aren't supposed to. So celebrate with the social network that helped you complete these four weeks. Throw a potluck with favorite Blue Zones meals you discovered throughout the past four weeks, or head on a walk together that ends at a great Wine @ 5 happy hour destination. Better yet: Hit a new milestone, literally, by tackling a longer walk your group has always wanted to achieve. Whatever you do, do it together and celebrate your success. Share a picture of your *moai* with #bluezoneslife on social media.

Keep Going

Continue to follow the sustainability plan on these next few pages. This is a lifestyle, not a diet or a short reset. To keep going for life, it has to be enjoyable. It shouldn't be a struggle. You should have found some plant-slant recipes you enjoy this month. Keep making the Blue Zones dishes you love and set out to discover more. Keep volunteering. Keep adding friends who share your passion for a healthy lifestyle to the mix. If you've struggled with any part of it—finding a group you like, recipes you love, or more friends with healthy lifestyles—that is okay. Keep trying and keep in mind that Rome wasn't built in a day.

REFLECTIONS

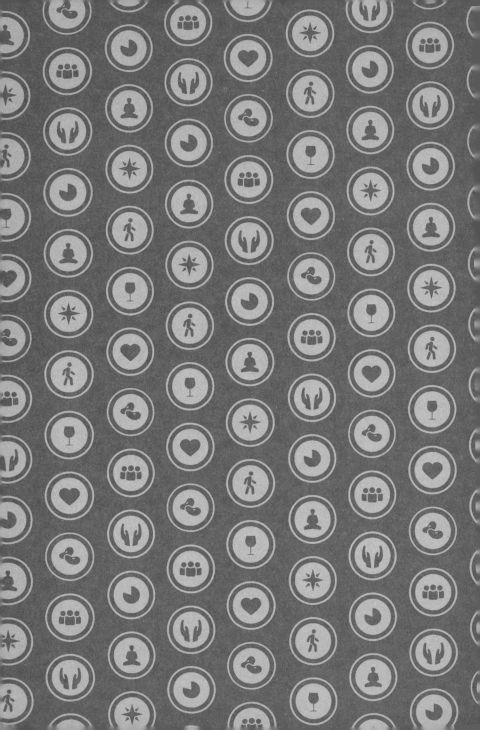

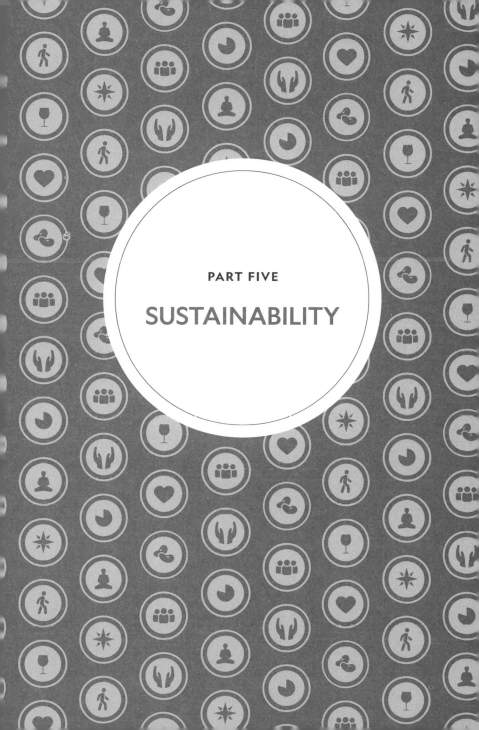

PART FIVE

SUSTAINABILITY

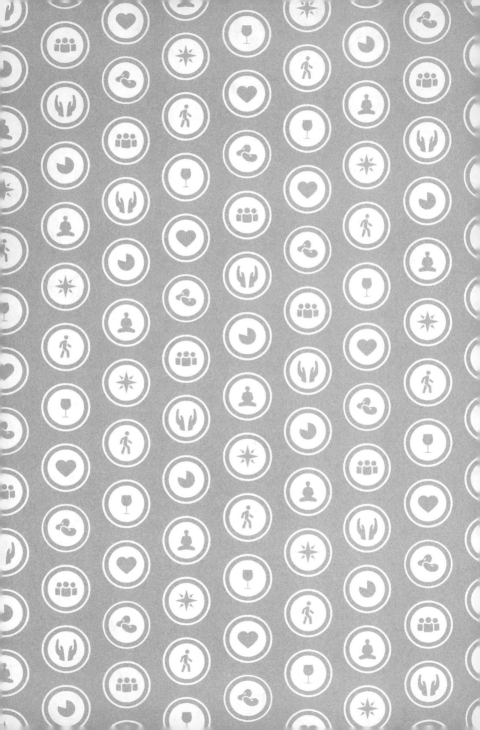

≈

Turn Your Challenge Into a Lifestyle

OW THAT YOU'VE FINISHED YOUR FOUR WEEKS OF THE BLUE ZONES CHALLENGE, you can use this planner for the rest of the year to reinforce what you've been learning and doing. Beyond just the benefit of tracking, we hope you get the emotional and mental boost that comes from writing and reflecting on your days, weeks, and years. These past four weeks are set up unlike any other program because we have trained you to start improving your environment and your social circle to influence the behavior and lifestyle changes you want. That's what we want you to stick with—not just eating one particular food (or not eating one food!) or doing one workout—but the practice of setting up your life to nudge you all day, every day, to achieve the life you want.

If your goals included losing weight, getting better sleep, or having more energy, then you will have already seen some of those changes. But more important, you are probably feeling the overall effects of this lifestyle, which can improve every aspect of your well-being from your mood to your energy to your productivity. You can adjust your goals along the way as you achieve or surpass them. But focus on the main objective, a better overall quality of life and more years of it, to stay on course for the rest of the year and the rest of your life—the joy of living a purpose-filled Blue Zones life.

REFLECTIONS

The Blue Zones Challenge
MONTH 2

Month 2 Activities

- Consider adopting a dog or a cat, if it fits your lifestyle.
- Hang light-blocking window shades in your bedroom to encourage better sleep.
- Continue the practice of *hara hachi bu* (stop eating when you're 80 percent full).
- Put indoor plants around your home.
- If you haven't already, enroll in an automatic savings or investment plan.
- Make a Sunday meal plan. Shop for your groceries and prep what you can for the week ahead.

3 Big Wins This Month

1. _____
2. _____
3. _____

Gratitude List

_____
_____
_____

Reflections

_____
_____
_____

THE BLUE ZONES CHALLENGE
MONTH 2 WORKSHEET

Day 1: _____

Day 2: _____

Day 3: _____

Day 4: _____

Day 5: _____

Day 6: _____

Day 7: _____

Day 8. _____

Day 9: _____

Day 10: _____

Day 11: _____

Day 12: _____

Day 13: _____

Day 14: _____

Day 15: _____

Day 16: _____

Day 17: _____

Day 18: _____

Day 19: _____

Day 20: _____

Day 21: _____

Day 22: _____

Day 23: _____

Day 24: _____

Day 25: _____

Day 26: _____

Day 27: _____

Day 28: _____

Day 29: _____

Day 30: _____

Day 31: _____

Service as the Antidote to Loneliness

I recently chatted with former surgeon general Dr. Vivek Murthy about his book *Together: The Healing Power of Human Connection in a Sometimes Lonely World.* Murthy teaches us that loneliness is a worldwide experience. In the United States, surveys indicate that at least 22 percent of adults struggle with loneliness. Many other countries have double-digit rates of loneliness, and it's affecting our health. Since loneliness triggers the stress response, chronic loneliness is akin to smoking 15 cigarettes a day and can lead to similar health issues like cancer, heart disease, and dementia.

In his book, Murthy identifies three types of loneliness: intimate, relational, and collective. Intimate loneliness is when we lack really close relationships with people who know us for our true selves. Relational loneliness is when we lack friendships—people we like to hang out with, confide in, or even go on vacation with. Finally, collective loneliness is the lack of a community-based or shared identity. We need to have all these types of connections, in balance, in our lives.

Building strong connections with others starts with building strong connections with ourselves, Murthy advocates. When we know and feel our value, we are confident and grounded. When we are lacking that self-confidence, we often go into a downward spiral. We think we're lonely because we're unlikable or we're not "good enough." This often gets even worse when we're bombarded with everybody else's "perfect" lives on social media.

The most profound antidote to loneliness, though, is through service. When we step out of our world and help others in need, we realize our value and build self-worth. It can be helping a neighbor who is struggling in isolation or collecting donations for a local shelter.

MONTH 2 REFLECTIONS

_____

_____

_____

_____

_____

_____

_____

_____

_____

_____

_____

_____

_____

_____

The Blue Zones Challenge
MONTH 3

Month 3 Activities

- Start a garden, whether in your yard, on your windowsill, or in an adopted plot at a local community garden.
- Designate a space in your home for quiet time, meditation, reading, or prayer.
- Set the temperature in your bedroom to 65 degrees Fahrenheit at night to encourage better sleep.
- Put a lavender plant next to your bed.
- Put a Post-it Note on your mirror with a reminder of your Purpose Statement. As an example, it might say "Grow and Give."

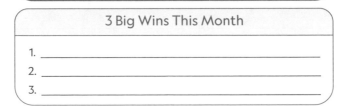

3 Big Wins This Month

1. _____
2. _____
3. _____

Gratitude List

_____
_____
_____

Reflections

_____
_____
_____

THE BLUE ZONES CHALLENGE
MONTH 3 WORKSHEET

Day 1: _____

Day 2: _____

Day 3: _____

Day 4: _____

Day 5: _____

Day 6: _____

Day 7: _____

Day 8: _____

Day 9: _____

Day 10: _____

Day 11: _____

Day 12: _____

Day 13: _____

Day 14: _____

Day 15: _____

Day 16: _____

Day 17: _____

Day 18: _____

Day 19: _____

Day 20: _____

Day 21: _____

Day 22: _____

Day 23: _____

Day 24: _____

Day 25: _____

Day 26: _____

Day 27: _____

Day 28: _____

Day 29: _____

Day 30: _____

Day 31: _____

Socialize More With the Right People

Research shows that friends and family can have a long-term impact on our health. In fact, if your best friends are obese, you're about twice as likely to be overweight. You are the sum of the people you spend the most time with, so spend some time optimizing your social circle for better health and happiness.

Americans had an average of three close friends in the 1980s. Today, that number has dropped to between one and two. If you don't have at least three friends whom you can call up on a bad day, research shows that you're shaving about eight years off your life expectancy.

In Okinawa, Japan, children were traditionally put into *moais*, groups of about five friends that have committed to one another for life. Most residents of Okinawa have *moais*, whether of their choosing or whether they were born into this type of close-knit community. Although the lifestyles of younger generations have changed in recent decades, some of the world's oldest women still live in Okinawa.

One particular *moai* that I discovered and spent some time with was made up of a group of women whose average age was 102. They got together every evening to drink sake and socialize.

Research shows that happiness is contagious, but so are smoking, obesity, and loneliness. The social circles of long-lived people have favorably shaped their health behaviors. To reap the benefits that blue zones residents experience, reach out more socially and nurture strong friendships. The more you socialize, the happier—and healthier—you'll be.

MONTH 3 REFLECTIONS

_____

_____

_____

_____

_____

_____

_____

_____

_____

_____

_____

_____

_____

_____

_____

_____

_____

The Blue Zones Challenge
MONTH 4

Month 4 Activities

- Try intermittent fasting and see how it works for you. Attempt to fast for 10 to 12 hours a few days a week.
- Spend at least one hour outside in nature (a city park counts), as many days as possible.
- If you find yourself having the urge to eat a snack, try drinking a whole glass of water slowly instead.
- Floss your teeth daily.
- Try a new Blue Zones recipe each week this month that includes an ingredient you've never cooked with before.
- Take time to declutter your home. Tackle one room per week.

3 Big Wins This Month

1. _____
2. _____
3. _____

Gratitude List

_____
_____
_____

Reflections

_____
_____
_____

THE BLUE ZONES CHALLENGE
MONTH 4 WORKSHEET

Day 1: _____

Day 2: _____

Day 3: _____

Day 4: _____

Day 5: _____

Day 6: _____

Day 7: _____

Day 8: _____

Day 9: _____

Day 10: _____

Day 11: _____

Day 12: _____

Day 13: _____

Day 14: _____

Day 15: _____

Day 16: _____

Day 17: _____

Day 18: _____

Day 19: _____

Day 20: _____

Day 21: _____

Day 22: _____

Day 23: _____

Day 24: _____

Day 25: _____

Day 26: _____

Day 27: _____

Day 28: _____

Day 29: _____

Day 30: _____

Day 31: _____

People of Faith Live Four to 14 Extra Years

Centenarians in blue zones regions are people of faith and take part in religious traditions and gatherings.

A study published in 2018 by the *Journal of the American Medical Association* is widely cited when it comes to women's longevity. Frequent organized religious attendance correlated with lower mortality in all categories, including from cancer and cardiovascular conditions. "Frequent" in this case was attending more than once a week, in comparison to those who did not attend at all. The women who attended more regularly had a 33 percent reduced chance of dying during the 16-year follow-up period than those who didn't.

A Vanderbilt University study of middle-age adults confirms this. Attending religious services regularly was linked to a 55 percent reduction in mortality for the 18-year follow-up period compared to individuals who did not attend services. The study also accounted for a stress index and found that there might be an independent effect of regular religious service attendance as it relates to mortality.

A longer-term study over 31 years showed similar results. The research aimed to look at the relationship between attending religious services and demographics, socioeconomic status, overall health, health behavior, and social networks. Scientists found that, consistent with most other research, religious attendance was correlated with longevity, as was high socioeconomic status.

This pattern emerges as we look more at the role religion plays in longevity. In a National Health Interview Survey, individuals who never attended some type of religious service were almost twice as likely to die in the follow-up period as those who attended more than once weekly. Interestingly, in this survey, individuals who attended services regularly were generally healthier than their peers, which would affect death rate. This survey also examined how religious attendance increased social networks, a factor that could also be at play.

MONTH 4 REFLECTIONS

_____

_____

_____

_____

_____

_____

_____

_____

_____

_____

_____

The Blue Zones Challenge
MONTH 5

Month 5 Activities

- Continue to walk at least once weekly with your group or walking buddy.
- Host a Blue Zones potluck once this month.
- Try a new Blue Zones recipe at least once a week.
- Take a 30-minute nap in the afternoon.
- Eat a light, early dinner. (Don't have a snack or dessert after!)
- Refill your countertop fruit bowl with seasonal fruits that you like.
- Review your Purpose Statement, and reflect on how you are living your purpose each day.

3 Big Wins This Month

1. _____
2. _____
3. _____

Gratitude List

_____
_____
_____

Reflections

_____
_____
_____

THE BLUE ZONES CHALLENGE MONTH 5 WORKSHEET

Day 1: _____

Day 2: _____

Day 3: _____

Day 4: _____

Day 5: _____

Day 6: _____

Day 7: _____

Day 8: _____

Day 9: _____

Day 10: _____

Day 11: _____

Day 12: _____

Day 13: _____

Day 14: _____

Day 15: _____

Day 16: _____

Day 17: _____

Day 18: _____

Day 19: _____

Day 20: _____

Day 21: _____

Day 22: _____

Day 23: _____

Day 24: _____

Day 25: _____

Day 26: _____

Day 27: _____

Day 28: _____

Day 29: _____

Day 30: _____

Day 31: _____

Fasting

Ikarians have traditionally been Greek Orthodox Christians, which means their religious calendar calls for fasting almost half of the year. Caloric restriction—a type of fasting that cuts about 30 percent of calories out of the normal diet—is the only proven way to slow the aging process in mammals.

A fast doesn't have to mean you stop eating for days. Instead, try to extend the time between your dinner and breakfast some days. If you eat dinner at 6 p.m. and breakfast at 8 a.m., then that's already a 14-hour fast.

MONTH 5 REFLECTIONS

_____

_____

_____

_____

_____

_____

_____

_____

_____

_____

_____

Checking In

You've now been following a Blue Zones lifestyle for four months after completing the challenge. Congratulate yourself on making this a sustainable, lifelong change. To be sure you're staying on track, make sure to do the following:

Retake the True Vitality Test (see page 66) and record your results.

True Vitality Score Week 1: _____

True Vitality Score Month 5: _____

Check in on your metrics: See the physical progress you've achieved over the past five months.

Metrics Checkup

Weight, Week 1: _____

Weight, Month 5: _____

BMI, Week 1: _____

BMI, Month 5: _____

Clothing Size, Week 1: _____

Clothing Size, Month 5: _____

Waist, Week 1: _____

Waist, Month 5: _____

- If your *moai* and Blue Zones buddy aren't working out, consider a refresh. Seek out a new Blue Zones buddy or join a different group. It's okay to find a new support system if the one you have isn't keeping you accountable and on track.

- Refresh your volunteering efforts—or find a way to give back if you aren't already.
- Celebrate your progress online. Use #bluezoneslife with pictures and posts on social media.
- Throw a celebratory Blue Zones potluck with your favorite foods from the past few months.
- Record how you're feeling, including your sense of purpose and progress in achieving your goals.

REFLECTIONS

_____
_____
_____
_____
_____
_____
_____
_____
_____
_____
_____
_____
_____
_____
_____
_____
_____
_____
_____
_____
_____
_____
_____
_____
_____
_____
_____
_____

The Blue Zones Challenge
MONTH 6

Month 6 Activities

- Continue to attend your groups, whether they are faith-based, social, or volunteer work.
- Create a Pride Shrine (bluezones.com/prideshrine) and update it with new achievements.
- Arrive at all your appointments this month 15 minutes early.
- Discover a new herbal tea that you love (p. 141).
- Don't eat any meals or snacks in front of the screen this month.
- Suggest and schedule a walking meeting at work.
- Limit your workweek to exactly 40 hours per week this month.

3 Big Wins This Month

1. _____
2. _____
3. _____

Gratitude List

_____
_____
_____

Reflections

_____
_____
_____

THE BLUE ZONES CHALLENGE
MONTH 6 WORKSHEET

Day 1: _____

Day 2: _____

Day 3: _____

Day 4: _____

Day 5: _____

Day 6: _____

Day 7: _____

Day 8: _____

Day 9: _____

Day 10: _____

Day 11: _____

Day 12: _____

Day 13: _____

Day 14: _____

Day 15: _____

Day 16: _____

Day 17: _____

Day 18: _____

Day 19: _____

Day 20: _____

Day 21: _____

Day 22: _____

Day 23: _____

Day 24: _____

Day 25: _____

Day 26: _____

Day 27: _____

Day 28: _____

Day 29: _____

Day 30: _____

Day 31: _____

Move Naturally, All Day

The world's longest-lived people don't pump iron, run marathons, or join gyms. Centenarians in the blue zones live in environments that nudge them to move naturally every 20 minutes, rather than separating fitness into a different part of their day. It's built into their lifestyles subconsciously.

If you look at how humans have evolved over time, they didn't sit down at a desk or on their couch for eight hours and then hope to make up for the inactivity with a half hour or 45 minutes in the gym. The way people live in the blue zones is an extension of how people have lived forever. Humans worked too hard for most of the history of our species and yet we have a natural inclination to want to rest. Now we also have technology and combustion engines to do a lot of our work for us. The sad by-product is that the work our bodies were engineered to do no longer gets done; our bodies don't get the regular low-intensity movement they need to thrive.

A study from the American Cancer Society followed 140,000 older adults and reported that those who walked six hours per week had a lower risk of dying from cardiovascular disease, respiratory disease, and cancer than those who were not active, but that walking even as little as two hours per week could begin to reduce the risk of disease and help you live a longer, healthier life.

A study of Amish communities in North America showed that the average woman logged 14,000 steps per day and the average man logged 18,000 steps per day, and both genders averaged about 10,000 steps on their day of rest. These Amish communities also had the lowest rates of obesity of any community in North America. This study eventually hit the media and began the movement to reach at least 10,000 steps per day.

Start moving naturally. Try "exercise snacks": In a study from the University of British Columbia, when, over a nine-hour period, overweight adults did a stair-climbing "exercise snack" every hour—briskly climbing 55 steps for about 20 seconds—their blood sugar levels were 17 percent lower than when they just spent the entire nine hours sitting.

MONTH 6 REFLECTIONS

_____

_____

_____

_____

_____

_____

_____

_____

_____

_____

The Blue Zones Challenge
MONTH 7

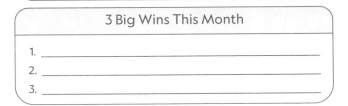

Month 7 Activities

- Review your Purpose Statement. Update it if you need to.
- Try meditation, yoga, or tai chi.
- Create a bedtime routine and stick with it.
- Volunteer for a cause about which you care deeply.
- Install a browser extension or app to remind you to stand or stretch every hour while at work or school (p. 142).
- Write a thank-you note to a co-worker or friend.
- Take time to rediscover a hobby you once loved.
- If you haven't already, start a container or outdoor garden (p. 181).

3 Big Wins This Month

1. _____
2. _____
3. _____

Gratitude List

_____
_____
_____

Reflections

_____
_____
_____

THE BLUE ZONES CHALLENGE MONTH 7 WORKSHEET

Day 1: _____

Day 2: _____

Day 3: _____

Day 4: _____

Day 5: _____

Day 6: _____

Day 7: _____

Day 0. _____

Day 9: _____

Day 10: _____

Day 11: _____

Day 12: _____

Day 13: _____

Day 14: _____

Day 15: _____

Day 16: _____

Day 17: _____

Day 18: _____

Day 19: _____

Day 20: _____

Day 21: _____

Day 22: _____

Day 23: _____

Day 24: _____

Day 25: _____

Day 26: _____

Day 27: _____

Day 28: _____

Day 29: _____

Day 30: _____

Day 31: _____

Moai Refresher

Moais are social groups of five to 10 people who gather together to share a common interest. The term *moai* ("mow-eye") comes from Okinawa, Japan, where people formed *moais* for life. This built-in social network guided them through good times and helped them through bad times. Social networks have a long-term, proven impact on health and well-being.

To create your own *moai*, follow these steps:

- Decide on a purpose or theme for your *moai*. It could be a walking *moai,* a potluck *moai* to share healthy recipes, or a knitting *moai.* Get creative. Think of an activity you enjoy that would allow for good conversation.
- Invite friends and family. Have them spread the word to extend your network.
- Plan to meet for 30 minutes at least once a week for 10 weeks and monitor your progress and mood.

MONTH 7 REFLECTIONS

The Blue Zones Challenge
MONTH 8

Month 8 Activities

- Make sure to have no more than one hour of additional screen time per day.
- Plan a future vacation (research confirms that taking a vacation could help you live longer).
- Make a plan to have lunch or coffee with a co-worker.
- Snack on nuts.
- Start a meditation practice, if you haven't already (p. 162).
- Try out a new faith-based organization if you're not already part of a spiritual community.
- Enjoy a Japanese or Costa Rican breakfast.
- Practice listening to someone with great attention.

3 Big Wins This Month

1. _____
2. _____
3. _____

Gratitude List

_____
_____
_____

Reflections

_____
_____
_____

THE BLUE ZONES CHALLENGE
MONTH 8 WORKSHEET

Day 1: _____

Day 2: _____

Day 3: _____

Day 4: _____

Day 5: _____

Day 6: _____

Day 7: _____

Day 8: _____

Day 9: _____

Day 10: _____

Day 11: _____

Day 12: _____

Day 13: _____

Day 14: _____

Day 15: _____

Day 16: _____

Day 17: _____

Day 18: _____

Day 19: _____

Day 20: _____

Day 21: _____

Day 22: _____

Day 23: _____

Day 24: _____

Day 25: _____

Day 26: _____

Day 27: _____

Day 28: _____

Day 29: _____

Day 30: _____

Day 31: _____

Power Foods to Boost Your Mood

Spinach

A significant source of vitamins K, A, and C, spinach is also an excellent source of folic acid, a B vitamin sometimes used to treat depression.

Oatmeal

High-fiber carbs like oatmeal stabilize blood sugar and take a while to move through your system, making you feel full longer.

Foods With Vitamin D

Getting some of your vitamin D (found in almond milk, oatmeal, fortified tofu, and orange juice) is important for your attitude.

Bananas

Bananas contain an amino acid called tryptophan. Your body uses tryptophan to produce 5-HTP, the compound that makes mood-boosting serotonin and melatonin.

Dark Chocolate

Eating chocolate releases serotonin and promotes relaxation through the release of endorphins.

MONTH 8 REFLECTIONS

The Blue Zones Challenge
MONTH 9

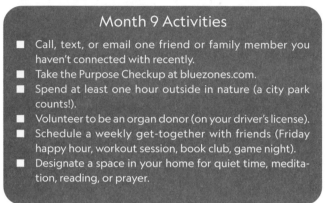

Month 9 Activities

- Call, text, or email one friend or family member you haven't connected with recently.
- Take the Purpose Checkup at bluezones.com.
- Spend at least one hour outside in nature (a city park counts!).
- Volunteer to be an organ donor (on your driver's license).
- Schedule a weekly get-together with friends (Friday happy hour, workout session, book club, game night).
- Designate a space in your home for quiet time, meditation, reading, or prayer.

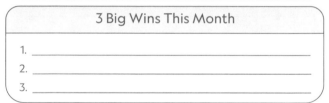

3 Big Wins This Month

1. _____
2. _____
3. _____

Gratitude List

_____
_____
_____

Reflections

_____
_____
_____

THE BLUE ZONES CHALLENGE
MONTH 9 WORKSHEET

Day 1: _____

Day 2: _____

Day 3: _____

Day 4: _____

Day 5: _____

Day 6: _____

Day 7: _____

Day 8: _____

Day 9: _____

Day 10: _____

Day 11: _____

Day 12: _____

Day 13: _____

Day 14: _____

Day 15: _____

Day 16: _____

Day 17: _____

Day 18: _____

Day 19: _____

Day 20: _____

Day 21: _____

Day 22: _____

Day 23: _____

Day 24: _____

Day 25: _____

Day 26: _____

Day 27: _____

Day 28: _____

Day 29: _____

Day 30: _____

Day 31: _____

Journaling

It turns out our dear diaries can be more than just a repository of our memories. Research from James Pennebaker, Ph.D., of the University of Texas at Austin, and Joshua Smyth, Ph.D., of Syracuse University has shown that writing about emotions can boost immune systems in patients with illnesses. In other research, it's also been effective in improving overall well-being in patients with anxiety and in improving working memory.

MONTH 9 REFLECTIONS

_____
_____
_____
_____
_____
_____
_____
_____
_____
_____
_____
_____
_____
_____
_____
_____
_____
_____
_____
_____
_____
_____
_____
_____
_____
_____
_____
_____

Checking In

You're almost to the one-year finish line, with nine months of the Blue Zones Challenge under your belt. Way to go! Don't forget to take the time to record your progress and reflect on the lifestyle changes you've made. Start thinking about how you will sustain a Blue Zones lifestyle in the years to come.

Retake the True Vitality Test (see page 66) and record your results.

True Vitality Score Week 1: _____

True Vitality Score Month 9: _____

Check in on your metrics: See the physical progress you've achieved over the past nine months.

Metrics Checkup

Weight, Week 1: _____

Weight, Month 9: _____

BMI, Week 1: _____

BMI, Month 9: _____

Clothing Size, Week 1: _____

Clothing Size, Month 9: _____

Waist, Week 1: _____

Waist, Month 9: _____

- If your *moai* and Blue Zones buddy aren't working out, consider a refresh. Seek out a new Blue Zones buddy or join a different group. It's okay to find a new support system if the one you have isn't keeping you accountable and on track.
- Refresh your volunteering efforts—or find a way to give back if you aren't already.
- Celebrate your progress online. Use #bluezoneslife with pictures and posts on social media.
- Throw a celebratory Blue Zones potluck with your favorite foods from the past few months.
- Record how you're feeling, including your sense of purpose and progress in achieving your goals.

REFLECTIONS

_____

_____

_____

_____

_____

_____

_____

_____

_____

_____

The Blue Zones Challenge
MONTH 10

Month 10 Activities

- Continue to practice *hara hachi bu* (stop eating when you are 80 percent full).
- Set a reminder or leave a note stuck to your fridge door to drink water throughout the day.
- Set the temperature in your bedroom to 65 degrees Fahrenheit at night to encourage better sleep.
- Take a 30-minute nap in the afternoon.
- Put your bike helmet or walking shoes by the door as a constant reminder for you to get up and get moving.
- Volunteer for a new organization.

3 Big Wins This Month

1. _____
2. _____
3. _____

Gratitude List

_____
_____
_____

Reflections

_____
_____
_____

THE BLUE ZONES CHALLENGE
MONTH 10 WORKSHEET

Day 1: _____

Day 2: _____

Day 3: _____

Day 4: _____

Day 5: _____

Day 6: _____

Day 7: _____

Day 8: _____

Day 9: _____

Day 10: _____

Day 11: _____

Day 12: _____

Day 13: _____

Day 14: _____

Day 15: _____

Day 16: _____

Day 17: _____

Day 18: _____

Day 19: _____

Day 20: _____

Day 21: _____

Day 22: _____

Day 23: _____

Day 24: _____

Day 25: _____

Day 26: _____

Day 27: _____

Day 28: _____

Day 29: _____

Day 30: _____

Day 31: _____

Gut Health

A healthy microbiome keeps *you* healthy, and it doesn't just affect your digestive system. The friendly bacteria found in your microbiome, or gut, are protective of everything from your risk of infection to your mood to your immune system.

You shouldn't have to rely on expensive supplements to improve your gut health. You can get many of the good bacteria your gut needs by changing aspects of your environment.

Six Ways to Improve Your Gut Health

- Eat more whole grains, nuts, veggies, beans, and fresh fruits.
- Brush and floss your teeth regularly. Studies at Cornell University and in Sweden have found that bacteria from your mouth can get into your stomach and cause problems.
- To improve good bacteria in your belly, eat fermented foods like sauerkraut, kefir, kimchi, kombucha, tempeh, and low-sugar yogurt.
- Eat foods rich in polyphenols like dark chocolate.
- Season with garlic, turmeric, and ginger to help rid your body of harmful bacteria.
- Limit artificial sweeteners.

MONTH 10 REFLECTIONS

The Blue Zones Challenge
MONTH 11

Month 11 Activities

- Continue to attend group gatherings.
- Continue to walk at least once weekly with others.
- Fill out a gratitude list each week.
- Turn off your devices at least one hour before bed.
- Make one new Blue Zones recipe this month.
- Get some sun, at least 15 minutes per day.
- Place cushions on the floor in your living room or office. Sit on the floor instead of the couch or chair while watching television or working (p. 114).
- Embrace your chores. Do yard work, cooking, and dishes entirely by hand.

3 Big Wins This Month

1. _____
2. _____
3. _____

Gratitude List

_____
_____
_____

Reflections

_____
_____
_____

THE BLUE ZONES CHALLENGE MONTH 11 WORKSHEET

Day 1: _____

Day 2: _____

Day 3: _____

Day 4: _____

Day 5: _____

Day 6: _____

Day 7: _____

Day 8: _____

Day 9: _____

Day 10: _____

Day 11: _____

Day 12: _____

Day 13: _____

Day 14: _____

Day 15: _____

Day 16: _____

Day 17: _____

Day 18: _____

Day 19: _____

Day 20: _____

Day 21: _____

Day 22: _____

Day 23: _____

Day 24: _____

Day 25: _____

Day 26: _____

Day 27: _____

Day 28: _____

Day 29: _____

Day 30: _____

Day 31: _____

Hara Hachi Bu

If you've ever been lucky enough to eat with an Okinawan elder, you've invariably heard them intone this Confucian-inspired adage before beginning the meal: *hara hachi bu*—a reminder to stop eating when their stomachs are 80 percent full. This cultural practice of calorie restriction (page 22) and mindful eating is part of the reason that Okinawa has a higher percentage of centenarians than anywhere else in the world.

Here's how you can practice *hara hachi bu* at home:

Eat more slowly.
Eating faster results in eating more. Slow down to allow your body to respond to cues, which tell us we are no longer hungry.

Focus on food.
Turn off the TV and the computer. If you're going to eat, just eat. You'll eat more slowly, consume less, and savor the food more.

Use smaller vessels.
Choose to eat on smaller plates and use tall, narrow glasses. You're likely to eat significantly less without even thinking about it.

MONTH 11 REFLECTIONS

The Blue Zones Challenge
MONTH 12

Month 12 Activities

■ Eat at least three Blue Zones meals every week.
■ Host a celebratory potluck to share your favorite recipes with your family or *moai*.
■ Limit your workweek to 40 hours.
■ Replenish the fruit bowl on your counter with seasonal and favorite fruits.
■ Volunteer for a new organization.
■ Call, text, or email one friend or family member you haven't connected with recently.
■ Write a thank-you note to a friend or co-worker—or even your Blue Zones buddy.

3 Big Wins This Month

1. _____
2. _____
3. _____

Gratitude List

_____
_____
_____

Reflections

_____
_____
_____

THE BLUE ZONES CHALLENGE
MONTH 12 WORKSHEET

Day 1: _____

Day 2: _____

Day 3: _____

Day 4: _____

Day 5: _____

Day 6: _____

Day 7: _____

Day 8: _____

Day 9: _____

Day 10: _____

Day 11: _____

Day 12: _____

Day 13: _____

Day 14: _____

Day 15: _____

Day 16: _____

Day 17: _____

Day 18: _____

Day 19: _____

Day 20: _____

Day 21: _____

Day 22: _____

Day 23: _____

Day 24: _____

Day 25: _____

Day 26: _____

Day 27: _____

Day 28: _____

Day 29: _____

Day 30: _____

Day 31: _____

Checking In
· ·

You did it! From the first four weeks of the challenge to the end of this month, you've completed one year of living the Blue Zones way. Take time to congratulate yourself, review your progress over the course of the year, and reflect on how the changes have impacted your life overall—from your health to your happiness.

Retake the True Vitality Test (see page 66) and record your results.
True Vitality Score Week 1: _____

True Vitality Score Month 12: _____

Retake the True Happiness Test (see page 71) and record your results.
True Happiness Score Week 1: _____

True Happiness Score Month 12: _____

Retake the Purpose Checkup (see page 76) and record your results.
Purpose Checkup Week 1: _____

Purpose Checkup Month 12: _____

Check in on your metrics: See the physical progress you've achieved over the past twelve months.

Metrics Checkup

Weight, Week 1: _____

Weight, Month 12: _____

BMI, Week 1: _____

BMI, Month 12: _____

Clothing Size, Week 1: _____

Clothing Size, Month 12: _____

Waist, Week 1: _____

Waist, Month 12: _____

Continue on from here. Now that you've made it a whole year, living a Blue Zones lifestyle should be second nature. Still, it's always good to check in from time to time and make sure you're staying on track. Don't forget to do the following:

- If your *moai* and Blue Zones buddy aren't working out, consider a refresh. Seek out a new Blue Zones buddy or join a different group. It's okay to find a new support system if the one you have isn't keeping you accountable and on track.
- Refresh your volunteering efforts—or find a way to give back if you aren't already.
- Celebrate your progress online. Use #bluezoneslife with pictures and posts on social media.
- Throw a celebratory Blue Zones potluck with your favorite foods from the past few months.
- Record how you're feeling, including your sense of purpose and progress in achieving your goals.

REFLECTIONS

REFLECTIONS

_____
_____
_____
_____
_____
_____
_____
_____
_____
_____
_____
_____
_____
_____
_____
_____
_____
_____
_____
_____
_____
_____
_____
_____

You Did It, Congrats!

Congratulations! You've finished the first year of the rest of your Blue Zones life. I hope you've reengineered your current surroundings and social circle to replicate the ancient practices we know support happier days and longer lives. I encourage you to keep tracking your days if you wish and to frequently measure where you stand on the True Vitality and True Happiness Tests. But I hope the biggest takeaway you get from this first year is that by setting up your life, social circle, and schedule to support the life you want, living the Blue Zones life is not a daily struggle but something that you wake up excited to do.

I consider it an honor and a privilege to bring this ancient wisdom to our modern lives, where many of us are stressed and sad. It takes all of us, many villages, to turn the tide. Thank you for coming along for the ride and for entrusting me with your time and energy.

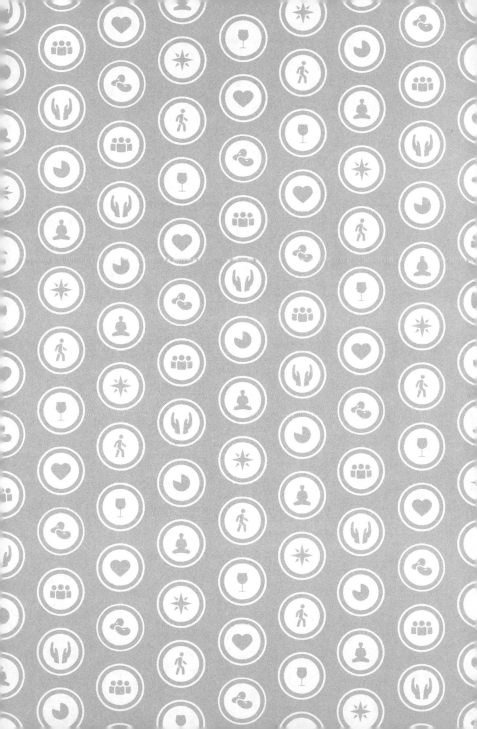

SOURCES

Make Movement Natural, pp. 111–117

Butryn, M. L., S. Phelan, J. O. Hill, and R. R. Wing. Consistent self-monitoring of weight: a key component of successful weight loss maintenance. *Obesity* 15, no. 12 (Dec. 2007):3091-6. doi: 10.1038/oby.2007.368. PMID: 18198319.

LaRose, J. G., A. Lanoye, D. F. Tate, and R. R. Wing. Frequency of self-weighing and weight loss outcomes within a brief lifestyle intervention targeting emerging adults. *Obes Sci Pract* 2, no. 1 (Mar. 2016):88-92. doi: 10.1002/osp4.24. Epub Feb. 19, 2016. PMID: 27668087; PMCID: PMC5021162.

O'Neil, P. M., and J. D. Brown. Weighing the evidence: benefits of regular weight monitoring for weight control. *J Nutr Educ Behav* 37, no. 6 (Nov.–Dec. 2005):319-22. doi: 10.1016/s1499-4046(06)60163-2. PMID: 16242064.

VanWormer, J. J., J. A. Linde, L. J. Harnack, S. D. Stovitz, and R. W. Jeffery. Self-weighing frequency is associated with weight gain prevention over 2 years among working adults. *Int J Behav Med* 19, no. 3 (Sept. 2012):351-8. doi: 10.1007/s12529-011-9178-1. PMID: 21732212

Why Record What You Eat?, p. 144

Ferrara, G., J. Kim, S. Lin, J. Hua, and E. Seto. A focused review of smartphone diet-tracking apps: usability, functionality, coherence with behavior change theory, and comparative validity of nutrient intake and energy estimates. *JMIR mHealth uHealth* 7, no. 5 (2019):e9232. Published May 17, 2019. doi:10.2196/mhealth.9232.

Harvey, J., R. Krukowski, J. Priest, and D. West. (2019), Log often, lose more: electronic dietary self-monitoring for weight loss. *Obesity*, 27, no. 27 (March 2019): 380-84. https://doi.org/10.1002/oby.22382.

Hollis, J. F., C. M. Gullion, V. J. Stevens, P. J. Brantley, L. J. Appel, J. D. Ard, C. M. Champagne, A. Dalcin, T. P. Erlinger, K. Funk, D. Laferriere,

P. H. Lin, C. M. Loria, C. Samuel-Hodge, W. M. Vollmer, and L. P. Svetkey; Weight Loss Maintenance Trial Research Group. Weight loss during the intensive intervention phase of the weight-loss maintenance trial. *Am J Prev Med* 35, no. 2 (Aug. 2008):118-26. doi: 10.1016/j.amepre.2008.04.013. PMID: 18617080; PMCID: PMC2515566.

Start a Meditation Practice, pp. 162–163

Chen, K.W., C. C. Berger, E. Manheimer, D. Forde, J. Magidson, L. Dachman, and C. W. Lejuez. Meditative therapies for reducing anxiety: a systematic review and meta-analysis of randomized controlled trials. *Depress Anxiety* 29, no. 7 (July 2012):545-62. doi: 10.1002/da.21964. Epub June 14, 2012. PMID: 22700446; PMCID: PMC3718554.

Gaylord, S. A., O. S. Palsson, E. L. Garland, K. R. Faurot, R. S. Coble, J. D. Mann, W. Frey, K. Leniek, and W. E. Whitehead. Mindfulness training reduces the severity of irritable bowel syndrome in women: results of a randomized controlled trial. *Am J Gastroenterol* 106, no. 9 (Sept. 2011):1678-88. doi: 10.1038/ajg.2011.184. Epub June 21, 2011. PMID: 21691341; PMCID: PMC6502251.

Goldstein, C. M., R. Josephson, S. Xie, and J. W. Hughes. Current perspectives on the use of meditation to reduce blood pressure. *Int J Hypertens* 2012;2012:578397. doi: 10.1155/2012/578397. Epub Mar. 5, 2012. PMID: 22518287; PMCID: PMC3303565.

Jedel, S., A. Hoffman, P. Merriman, B. Swanson, R. Voigt, K. B. Rajan, M. Shaikh, H. Li, and A. Keshavarzian. A randomized controlled trial of mindfulness-based stress reduction to prevent flare-up in patients with inactive ulcerative colitis. *Digestion* 89, no. 2 (2014):142-55. doi: 10.1159/000356316. Epub Feb. 14, 2014. PMID: 24557009; PMCID: PMC4059005.

Morgan, N., M. R. Irwin, M. Chung, and C. Wang. The effects of mind-body therapies on the immune system: meta-analysis. *PLOS One* 9, no. 7 (July 2014):e100903. doi: 10.1371/journal.pone.0100903. PMID: 24988414; PMCID: PMC4079606.

Ong, J. C., R. Manber, Z. Segal, Y. Xia, S. Shapiro, and J. K. Wyatt. A randomized controlled trial of mindfulness meditation for chronic insomnia. *Sleep* 37, no. 9 (Sept. 2014):1553-63. doi: 10.5665/sleep.4010. PMID: 25142566; PMCID: PMC4153063.

Sleep, pp. 184–185

Al-Abri, M. A. Sleep deprivation and depression: A bi-directional association. *Sultan Qaboos Univ Med J* 15, no. 1 (2015):e4-e6.

Worley, S. L., The extraordinary importance of sleep: the detrimental effects of inadequate sleep on health and public safety drive an explosion of sleep research. *P T* 43, no. 12 (2018):758-63.

People of Faith Live Four to 14 Extra Years, pp. 208–209

Bruce, M. A., D. Martins, K. Duru, B. M. Beech, M. Sims, et al. Church attendance, allostatic load and mortality in middle aged adults. *PLOS One* 12, no. 5 (2017): e0177618.

Hummer, R. A., R. G. Rogers, C. B. Nam, and C. G. Ellison. Religious involvement and U.S. adult mortality. *Demography* 36, no. 2 (May 1999):273-85. PMID: 10332617.

Acknowledgments

This book would not have been possible without the help of many.

The insight—change your surroundings, not your environment—came from two men. The first, Pekka Puska, ran the first measurably successful population health project in North Karelia, Finland. His project was a prototype–Blue Zones Project of sorts. And Ikarian Stamitis Moriatis, who when I asked how he managed to live to 102 after a terminal lung cancer diagnosis at age 66, said, "I don't know, I just forgot to die."

Of the dozens of scientists I've worked with, first thanks goes to Dr. Gianni Pes, who not only identified Sardinia's blue zones region but, nearly two decades later, continues to mine insights for the world on living longer, better. He serves as chief scientific consultant as well as a guide in the Sardinian blue zones region. He, along with demographer Michel Poulain, helped me identify Nicoya, Costa Rica; Ikaria, Greece; and Okinawa, Japan, as blue zones.

From the Blue Zones team, my thanks goes to Naomi Imatome-Yun for her work editing this book and pulling it all together. At National Geographic, I thank editorial director and publisher Lisa Thomas, who has commissioned every Blue Zones book and orchestrated each one's success. And to the editorial team—senior editor Allyson Johnson, designer Lisa Monias, art director Sanaa Akkach, and senior production editor Judith Klein—I am deeply grateful for your work and dedication to this book.

My superb team back at Blue Zones headquarters includes Amelia Clabots, Aislinn Leonard, Souraya Farhat, and my Right-Hand Man, Sam Skemp.

About the Author

Dan Buettner is the founder of Blue Zones, an organization that helps Americans live longer, healthier, happier lives. His groundbreaking work on longevity led to his 2005 *National Geographic* cover story: "The Secrets of Long Life" and four national bestsellers: *The Blue Zones, Thrive, The Blue Zones Solution,* and *The Blue Zones Kitchen.* He is also the author of *The Blue Zones of Happiness.* He lives in Miami, Florida. Find him on Instagram (@danbuettner) and at danbuettner.com.

Learn more about the Blue Zones on Facebook (facebook.com/BlueZones) and Twitter and Instagram (@BlueZones), and at bluezones.com.

Since 1888, the National Geographic Society has funded more than 14,000 research, conservation, education, and storytelling projects around the world. National Geographic Partners distributes a portion of the funds it receives from your purchase to National Geographic Society to support programs including the conservation of animals and their habitats.

Get closer to National Geographic Explorers and photographers, and connect with our global community. Join us today at nationalgeographic .com/join

For rights or permissions inquiries, please contact National Geographic Books Subsidiary Rights: bookrights@natgeo.com

The Purpose Checkup and Purpose Statement on pages 76-82 from "A Guide to Unlocking the Power of Purpose" by Richard Leider, used with permission.

ISBN: 978-1-4262-2194-1

Printed in the United States of America

21/WOR/2

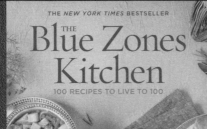
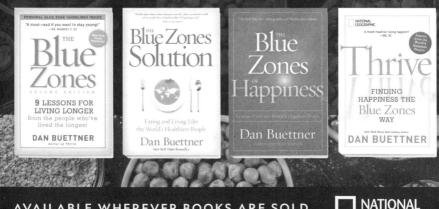